Palokinam PITCHE

SEXUALLY TRANSMITTED INFECTIONS

Palokinam PITCHE

SEXUALLY TRANSMITTED INFECTIONS

From the clinic to public health

ScienciaScripts

Imprint
Any brand names and product names mentioned in this book are subject to trademark, brand or patent protection and are trademarks or registered trademarks of their respective holders. The use of brand names, product names, common names, trade names, product descriptions etc. even without a particular marking in this work is in no way to be construed to mean that such names may be regarded as unrestricted in respect of trademark and brand protection legislation and could thus be used by anyone.

Cover image: www.ingimage.com

This book is a translation from the original published under ISBN 978-620-6-70354-9.

Publisher:
Sciencia Scripts
is a trademark of
Dodo Books Indian Ocean Ltd. and OmniScriptum S.R.L publishing group

120 High Road, East Finchley, London, N2 9ED, United Kingdom
Str. Armeneasca 28/1, office 1, Chisinau MD-2012, Republic of Moldova, Europe
Printed at: see last page
ISBN: 978-620-7-61139-3

Contents

Preface

Sexually transmitted infections (1ST) are a global public health problem, with higher occurrences in certain regions such as sub-Saharan Africa and Latin America, and in certain at-risk groups.
Knowledge and treatment of STIs have progressed considerably in recent decades thanks to the dynamism of scientific research in the fight against the HIV epidemic.
In epidemiological terms, we have recently seen the emergence of new STIs (Zika virus, Ebola virus, monkeypox virus). The problem of managing them is marked by the continuing and growing resistance of certain bacterial agents such as Neisseria gonorrheae and Mycoplasma genitalium to antibiotics.
Management of 1ST must be comprehensive. It covers diagnosis, treatment of the patient, risk reduction for the patient, and breaking the chain of transmission by caring for sexual partners. For this care to be effective and efficient, STIs must be integrated into the general framework of sexual and reproductive health, taking into account all the issues relating to the right to health and gender-based violence, which increase the vulnerability of women and girls to these diseases. In addition, effective treatment of STIs is still hampered by a lack of technical facilities and qualified personnel, as well as financial and geographical difficulties in accessing appropriate care in countries with limited resources.
This book is a comprehensive guide to the management of STIs. It covers not only the purely medical aspects, with an update of scientific data taking account of the main diagnostic and therapeutic advances, but also the public health perspective, with chapters on syndromic management and standards and procedures for service provision.
Professor PITCHE has extensive experience and expertise both as a clinician and as a manager of STI/HIV programmes. His experience explains the high quality of this book, which is aimed at medical students, practising health professionals and public health workers.

Mrs Kissem TCHANGAI-WALLA

Honorary Professor of Dermato-Venereology at the University of Lome
Former Minister for Social Affairs and the Civil Service

Foreword

Sexually transmitted infections (STIs) or sexually transmitted diseases (STDs) are common ailments and a public health problem because of their morbidity in young people, particularly in the context of the HIV epidemic.

The management of STIs is a practical challenge for all clinicians, who need to be familiar with the symptoms of each condition and the appropriate diagnostic approach to follow. The clinical and etiological spectrum of 1STs has become quite broad in recent years. In fact, alongside the classic 1STs such as gonorrhoea, chlamydia, trichomoniasis, herpes and condylomata, we are seeing emerging or re-emerging STIs. Some STIs, such as chancroid and donovanosis, have become very rare or are in the process of being eliminated.

In recent years, the growing development of rapid molecular biology diagnostic techniques (point-of-care tests) that do not require expensive technical facilities has made these diagnostic methods more accessible in most countries. The therapeutic management of these conditions is dynamic, taking into account the ongoing development of antibiotic resistance in certain bacterial STIs.

Effectively combating STIs has been a public health issue for several years now. The clinician must therefore manage the patient (and not the disease), taking account of the patient's individuality. However, both clinicians and programme managers need to integrate this care into a virtuous circle that places the target population at the centre of their activities. In fact, the management of STIs must be holistic and tailored to each population group, which varies according to the social and epidemiological context. This obliges all stakeholders to put in place strategies to provide quality services covering the entire spectrum of the fight against these diseases, from prevention to optimal therapeutic care for patients and their sexual partners. Any health programme must therefore guarantee a minimum quality of service that is effective and acceptable to the target population, at all levels of care.

The aim of this book is to provide healthcare providers with an up-to-date working tool covering all aspects of STIs. It is also adapted to all conditions of practice, particularly in countries with limited resources. The main therapeutic strategies have been updated and are based on scientific evidence and the latest international recommendations on the subject.

Palokinam PITCHE

Acknowledgements

To Dr Y. Kelem for reading the document and to Mrs Solange Poidy for her invaluable secretarial assistance.

PART I

I. Epidemiology and anatomical background

1. Epidemiology

Sexually transmitted infections (STIs) are diseases transmitted through unprotected sexual contact with a person who is already infected. This sexual contact occurs either between people of different sexes (heterosexual relations) or between people of the same sex (homosexual relations). There are a variety of possible contaminating sexual relations: the most common are purely genital relations (vaginal coitus, anal coitus), but there may also be relations involving oral-genital contact (fellatio, cunis lingus) or even simple physical contact, as is the case with the transmission of scabiosis and pediculosis [1-3].

Sexually transmitted infections (1ST) are a public health problem because of their prevalence and morbidity. Most of these infections lead to serious reproductive health complications, some of which are fatal (HIV infection, syphilis, cancers caused by human papillomavirus or hepatitis B and C viruses) [2-4].

Frequency

In 2018, the World Health Organisation (WHO) estimated that there were 376 million cases of curable STIs worldwide [5].

Table 1: Number of curable STI cases according to the WHO

Types of STI	**Number (millions)**
Gonorrhoea	87
Chlamydia	127
Trichomoniasis	156
Syphilis	06
Total	**376**

Between 1990 and 2019, trends have shown a significant decline in the incidence of curable STIs in the general population worldwide, particularly in northern countries, but in southern countries (sub-Saharan Africa, Latin America) the decline is less marked [6, 7]. Declines in incidence are linked to the prevention programmes, active testing and promotion of behavioural change that have been put in place in most countries with the advent of HIV infection. According to WHO reports, infections with chlamydia, gonococcus and syphilis are still prevalent in sub-Saharan Africa and Latin America [5].

The frequency of *Chlamydia trachomatis (CT)* infection is one of the major factors in infertility in young women [8, 9]. The incidence of CT is underestimated in most countries, because it is often asymptomatic or paucisymptomatic, especially in women, but also in men, which is a factor in the spread of the infection.

In Europe and the United States, certain population groups are significantly more affected by STIs [10, 11]. There has been a marked increase in gonococcal and syphilis infections among men who have sex with men (MSM) over the last twenty years [11-14]. The resurgence of syphilis is particularly marked among men who have sex with men (MSM) and people living with HIV [12]. In the United States, more than 58% of syphilis cases in 2016 were among MSM [10]. In some states in the southern United States, the incidence of syphilis doubled between 2014 and 2018 among heterosexual men and pregnant women in the Latin American and African-American groups [11]. Lymphogranulomatosis venereum, which had virtually disappeared in Europe in the 1970s and 1980s, re-emerged in all northern countries in the early 2000s [15, 16].

Being chronic infections, it is difficult to estimate the incidence of genital herpes and human papillomavirus genital infection. The WHO estimated the number of these two infections at 271 million in 2016, demonstrating their importance among 1ST [5]. The frequency of these two infections is even higher in HIV-infected and immunocompromised patients. Epidemiological data on the incidence of HPV infections in immunocompetent patients are not available. The rate of subclinical HPV carriage is estimated at 15%, and asymptomatic carriage is thought to be close to 100%, particularly in women [17].

Data on chancre mou and donovanosis are very patchy. In fact, these infections are typically found in tropical countries, and the majority of cases diagnosed in northern countries are imported. It is estimated that chancre mellitus is on the verge of extinction in certain African countries because of the sharp fall in its incidence over the last 20 years in healthcare centres [18].

Factors in the spread of STIs

The factors contributing to the spread of the disease are essentially linked to risky sexual behaviour (multiple sexual partners, failure to use condoms with occasional partners, underestimation of personal risk, sexual violence). In some groups, sexual behaviour is relaxed because of drug and alcohol use. With the introduction of antiretroviral drugs, HIV-seropositive MSM have been found to take greater risks than seronegative MSM [13, 14]. In some people on effective antiretroviral drugs, there is also a false assurance of non-contamination, which encourages risk-taking through unprotected sex. During the use of pre-exposure prophylaxis, the incidence of syphilis, gonorrhoea and chlamydia has been reported [17, 18]. In southern countries, risk behaviour in the heterosexual population is often linked to ignorance of the means of propagation and difficulties in accessing preventive measures such as the use of condoms (considered to be a contraceptive against pregnancy and opposed during the HIV pandemic by certain religious circles). There are also socio-economic vulnerability factors that often expose young girls and women to STIs and HIV. The social vulnerabilities of women in developing countries include all forms of gender-based violence (sexual violence, difficulty in negotiating the use of condoms by one's sexual partner, early or forced marriages, levirate and sororate practices) [19]. Economic vulnerability is linked to the financial difficulties of accessing quality health centres for screening and treatment of STI cases in order to cut the transmission chains. In addition, the phenomenon of transaction during sexual relations, in certain unfavourable socio-economic and political situations (such as wars and displacement as internal or external refugees) are particularly significant vulnerability factors for adolescent girls and women.

Morbidity factors

- *The problem of germ resistance to antibiotics*

Germ resistance to antibiotics is a public health issue. Surveillance of strains of NG resistant to antibiotics shows an increasing number of different classes of drugs that have become ineffective in the treatment of gonococcal disease [19-21]. This raises the problem of the availability of these drugs in the therapeutic armoury and in the definition of strategies for managing the infection. This phenomenon is beginning to be observed for agents such as *Mycoplasma genitallium and Chlamydia trachomatis* with macrolides.

- *Risk of infertility.*

This risk is not always easy to assess in a young woman with primary or secondary sterility, as the infectious episodes that have affected the uterine tubes and caused stenosis preventing the normal passage of the ovum are often several years old. Some 45-75% of secondary sterilisations in certain southern countries are due to pelvic inflammatory syndromes, which are regional complications of vaginal and cervical infections with *Neisseria gonorrhoeae* or *Chlamydia trachomatis* [17]. Gonococcal salpingitis tends to produce acute symptoms, which is not often the case with salpingitis due to *Chlamydia trachomatis* infection. *Chlamydia trachomatis* infections are unrecognised and therefore under-diagnosed, and are particularly dangerous because they develop quietly over several months or years, leading to inflammatory lesions of the fallopian tubes that can result in permanent obstruction. PID accounts for 20-44% of hospital admissions to obstetrics and gynaecology departments in developing countries [22-26]. The risk of infertility and sterility is generally underestimated in men (whatever the primary or secondary cause). STIs are one of the causes of secondary infertility in men. Orchiepididymitis with stenosis of the vas deferens can lead to oligospermia. Cases of chronic prostatitis and post-infectious urethral stenosis have been described [27].

- *Neonatal risk.*

Most 1ST are transmissible from mother to child. A woman with untreated gonococcal infection during pregnancy is thought to infect her child in 35-45% of cases [24]. The result will be severe neonatal gonococcal conjunctivitis, which may be complicated by corneal lesions (keratitis) leading to permanent blindness. This risk is lower when the mother is infected with *Chlamydia trachomatis* (32% of cases, with less aggressive conjunctivitis). Other consequences include prematurity, low birth weight, severe pulmonary infections, severe encephalitis in neonatal herpes and syphilis, and microcephaly in Zika virus infection [28]. In developing countries, the prevalence of congenital syphilis is estimated at between 4 and 20% [5]. A mother infected with syphilis has only one chance in three of giving birth to a healthy child. In 2018, according to WHO estimates, congenital syphilis is still a public health problem in Africa and the Americas. Between 2016 and 2017, the estimated number of cases of congenital syphilis per 100,000 live births was 48.9 in the African region and 28.9 in the Americas, compared with 0.4 in Europe. The morbidity of neonatal syphilis in southern countries has prompted the WHO to launch a global plan to eliminate congenital syphilis by 2030 [5].

- *Risk of contracting a severe or serious illness*

Rectitis in lymphogranulomatosis venereum can become chronic and stenosing. Gonococcal sepsis can be life-threatening and fatal. Certain *N. meningitidis* infections can lead to a systemic picture of meningitis which, if left untreated, can be fatal [23]. In the course of tertiary syphilis, death may occur, particularly in the case of destructive lesions of the aorta (aneurysm, aortitis) or severe neurological symptoms with meningitis, hemiplegia or terminal dementia [24]. Infection with viral hepatitis B and C can lead to cirrhosis and cancer [29]. The occurrence of cervical cancers in *Papillomavirus* infections is well documented [30,31].

- *Risk of HIV infection.*

The emergence of the HIV pandemic has overturned the "traditionally benign" concept of STIs. Sexual transmission accounts for 70-90% of HIV transmission [32, 33]. The virus is frequently found in semen and vaginal and cervical secretions. Any break in the mechanical barrier represented by a healthy mucosa favours HIV transmission. A genital ulcer, for example, increases the risk of HIV transmission by a factor of three to seven. All STIs that cause inflammation of the genital mucosa favour this transmission. In total, all STIs (ulceration or urethritis) favour HIV transmission, making STI patients a high-risk group.

The main micro-organisms responsible for STIs.

There are a great many of them, which explains the polymorphism of STIs. There are several types of germ (bacteria, viruses, parasites, fungi) that can be transmitted by sexual contact *(Tab. 2)*.

Table 2: Microorganisms responsible for 1ST [34].

Clinical syndromes	**Germs**
Genital discharge	*Neisseria gonorrheae* *Neisseria meningitidis* *Chiamedia tsouhoeatis (D to K strain)* *Vaichamonas vaginalis* *Gardnerellv vaginalis* *Mycoplasma hominis* *Mycoplasma genitalium Ureaplasma urealyticum Candida sp*
Genital ulcers	*Treponema pallidum subsp. Pallidum* *Haemophilus ducreyi* *Chlamydia trachomatis (serovars L1 L2 L3)* *Klebsiella granulomatis*

	Herpes simplex virus 1 and 2
Digestive syndromes (congestion, colitis, proctitis) or epilepsy	Hepatitis viruses A, B, C *Chlamydia traohomatis (sercwars L1 L2 L3) phigella sp* *Escherichia coli Campylobacter sp Entamoeba histolytica*
Systemic syndrome	*Treponema pallidum sbsp. pallidum N&sseria meningitidls (encapsule)* Zika virus Ebola virus *Pox virus*
Other syndromes	Human papilloma virus (HPV) *Sarcoptes scabei hominis* Phtirius pubis MCV (pox virus) HIV

References

1. Siboulet A, Coulaud JB. Sexually transmitted diseases. Abreges. 2ed Ed Masson 1991
2. Janier M. Maladies sexuellement transmissibles, collection Abrege. Masson-Elsevier 2010
3. Herida M, Michel A, Goulet V et al. The epidemiology of sexually transmitted infections in France. Med Mal Infect 2005; 35: 281-289
4. Landovitz RJ, Tseng CH, Weissman M et al. Epidemiology, sexual risk behavior, and HIV prevention practices of men who have sex with men using GRINDR in Los Angeles, California. J Urban Health 2013;90:729-39
5. World Health Organization. Global health sector strategy against sexually transmitted infections.
Https//:apps.who.int/bitstream/handle/10665/250242/WHO-RHR-169
6. Kularatne RS, Nil R, Rowley J et al. Adult gonorrhea, chlamydia and syphilis prevalence, incidence and syndromic case reporting in South Africa. PloS One 2018; 13 (10) e205863 Epub 2018 Oct 5
7. Neuman L, Rowley J, Vander-Hoom S et al. Global estimates of prevalence and incidence of curable sexually transmitted infections in 2012 based on systematic review of global reporting. PloS One 2015 (12) e143304 epu 2015 Dec 8
8. Rowley J, Vander-hoom S, Korenromp E et al. Chlamydia, gonorrheae, trichomiasis and syphilis. Global prevalence and incidence estimates. Bull Word health Organ 2019; 97: 548562
9. Stary A. The changing spectrum of Sexually transmitted infections in Europe. Acta Derm Venereol 2020 Mar 24. doi: 10.2340/00015555-3470.
10. Abara WE, Hess KL, Neblett Fanfair R et al. Syphilis Trends among men who have sex with men in the United States and Western Europe: A Systematic Review of Trend Studies Published between 2004 and 2015. PLoS One 2016; 11: e0159309
11. Hope-Rapp E, Anyfantakis V, Fouere S et al. Etiology of genital ulcer disease. A prospective study of 248 cases in Paris. Sex Transm Dis 2010;37:153-8.
12. Bernstein KT, Stephens SC, Strona FV et al. Epidemiologic characteristics of an ongoing syphilis epidemic among men who have sex with men, San Francisco. Sex Transm Dis 2013;40:11-7.
13. Kularatne RS, Muller EE, Maseko DV et al.Trends in the relative prevalence of genital ulcer disease pathogens and association with HIV infection in Johannesburg, South Africa, 2007-2015. PLoS One2018 Apr 4;13 (4):e0194125.doi: 10.1371/journal.pone.0194125. eCollection 2018.
14. Chow EPF, Grulich AE, Fairley CK. Epidemiology and prevention of sexually transmitted infections in men who have sex with men at risk of HIV.
Lancet HIV 2019;6:e396-e405. doi: 10.1016/S2352-3018(19)30043-8.
15. Zheng Y, Yu Q, Lin Y et al. Global burden and trends of sexually transmitted infections from 1990 to 2019: an observational trend study. Lancet Infect Dis. 2022 22:541-551.

16. Allawela SNS, Sullivan AK, Macdonald N et al. Clinical predictors of rectal lymphogranuloma venereum infection: results from a multicenter case-control study in the UK. Sex Transm Infect 2014,90:2674.
17. Unemo M, Bradshaw CS, Hocking JS et al. Sexually transmitted infections: challenges ahead.Lancet Infect Dis. 2017;17:e235-e279. doi: 10.1016/S1473-3099(17)30310-9.
18. Spiteri G, Unemo M, Mardh O et al. The resurgence of syphilis in high-income countries in the 2000s: a focus on Europe. Epidemiol Infect 2019;147:e143
19. Unemo M, Golparian D, Nicholas R et al. High-level cefixime and ceftriaxone-resistant Neisseria gonorrhoeae in France: novel penA mosaic allele in a successful international clone causes treatment failure. Antimicrob Agents Chemother 2012; 56:1273-80
20. Forsyth S, Penney P, Rooney G. Cefixime-resistant Neiseria gonorrhoeae in the UK: a time to reflect on practice and recommendations. Int J STD AIDS 2011 ;2 ; 296-7
21. Lewis DA, Sriruttan C, Muller EE et al. Phenotypic and genetic characterization of the first two cases of extended-spectrum-cephalosporin-resistant Neisseria gonorrhoeae in South Africa and association with cefixime treatment failure. J Antimicrob Chemother 2013; 68:1267-70
22. Tsevat DG, Wiesenfeld HC, David C et al Sexually transmitted diseases and infertility. Am J Obstet Gynecol 2017; 16:1-9.
23. Pellati D, Mylonakis I, Bertolon G et al. Genital tract infections and infertility Eur J Obstet Gynecol Reprod Biol 2008;140:3-11.
24. Moodley P, A W Sturm AW. Sexually transmitted infections, adverse pregnancy outcome and neonatal infection. Semin Neonatol 2000;5:255-69.
25. Lemly D, Gupta N. Sexually Transmitted Infections Part 2: Discharge Syndromes and Pelvic Inflammatory Disease. Pediatr Rev. 2020;41:522-537.
26. Shroff S. Infectious Vaginitis, Cervicitis, and Pelvic Inflammatory Disease. Med Clin North Am. 2023;107:299-315.
27. Spornraft-Ragaller P, Varwig-JanBen D. Sexually transmitted infections and male fertility. Hautarzt. 2018; 69:1006-1013.
28. Moreira J, Peisoto TM, Siquiera AM et al. Sexually acquired Zika virus: a systematic review. Clin Microbiol Infect 2017;23 :296-305
29. Alberts CJ, Clifford GM, Damien-Georges D et al. Worldwide prevalence of hepatitis B virus and hepatitis C virus among patients with cirrhosis at country, region, and global levels: a systematic review.Lancet Gastroenterol Hepatol 2022;7:724-735.
30. Rahangdale L, MungoSio C, O'Connor B et al. Human papillomavirus vaccination and cervical cancer risk. BMJ 2022;379:e070115. doi: 10.1136/bmj-2022-070115.
31. Martel C, Georges D, Bray F et al. Global burden of cancer attributable to infections in 2018: a worldwide incidence analysis. Lancet Glob Health. 2020;8:e180-e190. doi: 10.1016/S2214-109X(19)30488-7. Epub 2019 Dec 17.

2. Anatomical reminder of the genitalia

The anatomical site of 1ST is preferably the urogenital tract in men, and the genital tract in women. In order to understand the dynamics of these infections (transmission, clinical manifestations and possible complications), it is important to understand the anatomy of the genital systems of both sexes [1-3].

Male genitalia *(fig. 1 and 2)*

- *The ureter*

It starts at the neck of the bladder and ends at the urinary bladder, measuring 16 to 17 cm in length. It comprises the posterior and anterior urethra.

The first part of the posterior urethra is surrounded by the prostate, into which the ejaculatory ducts drain. The posterior urethra crosses the prostate from its base to its apex. The prostatic urethra is linked to the seminiferous vesicles which empty into the vas deferens. The posterior segment of the prostatic urethra therefore represents the crossroads of the urinary and genital tracts. Infection can occur via the ascending route following previous urethritis, or via the descending route following an upper urinary tract infection unrelated to an STI. The other part of the prostate urethra is the membranous urethra, which represents the lower part of the urethra. It is surrounded by striated muscle fibres, an expansion of the levator ani muscles. The anterior urethra forms the bulbar and perineal urethra. The bulbar urethra contains Cowper's glands, which can be infected by any infectious agent. When the urethra emerges from the pelvis and penetrates the penis, it is completely surrounded by the corpus spongiosum up to the level of the glans. The corpus spongiosum is surrounded laterally by two corpora cavernosa. The terminal part of the penile urethra contains submucosal glands known as Littre's glands, which can become infected.

- The *testicles* and *epididymis*

These are sperm-producing organs and are located under the penis, in the bursa. The epididymis lies on the upper edge of the testicle and the adjacent part of the outer surface of the testicle. The epididymis consists of three parts: the head, the body and the tail. The maximum lesions occur at the tail of the epididymis, where it terminates in the vas deferens. In the case of STIs, the testicle alone may be affected (orchitis) and/or associated with that of the epididymis (epididymitis) and may be the source of infertility in men. The vas deferens follows the tail of the epididymis and ends at the junction of the seminiferous vesicle and the ejaculatory duct.

Female urethro-genital system *(fig. 3)*

- *The urethra.* It is much shorter (3 to 4 cm). It follows on from the vesical neck and has a narrower and less dilatable meat than that of the man. This meat is located at the top and front of the vulva and sometimes ends in the front of the vagina, which may explain bacterial transmission from the vagina to the urethra during intercourse. Skene's paraurethral glands are located on either side of the urethra and drain into the lips.
- The *vagina* is a tube that runs from the cervix to the vulva. It lies in front of the rectum, behind the bladder and below the uterus. The end of the vagina opens into the vestibule.
- *The vulva* is the female external genitalia. It is bounded laterally by two juxtaposed folds of skin: the large lip to the outside and the small lip to the inside. Bartholin's glands are buried deep in the labia majora and are subject to acute or chronic infection.
- *The uterus.* This is a smooth, hollow musculus in the shape of a truncated cone, flattened from front to back. Its lower part, represented by the cervix, is cylindrical. The cervix projects into the vagina. The body is bordered at the top by two internal horns, where the fallopian tubes are implanted. The fallopian tubes are connected to the ovaries, which they cover with a pinna. Ligaments connect the ovary to neighbouring organs.

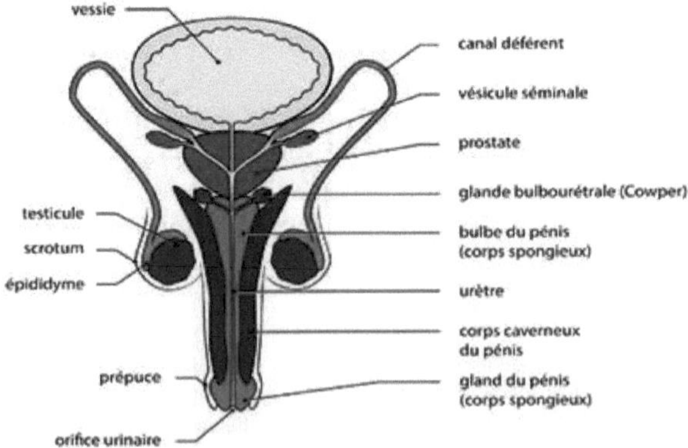

Figure 1: Anatomy of the male genitourinary organs (Front)

https://microbiologiemedicale.fr/anatomie-physiologie-appareil-genital-masculin/

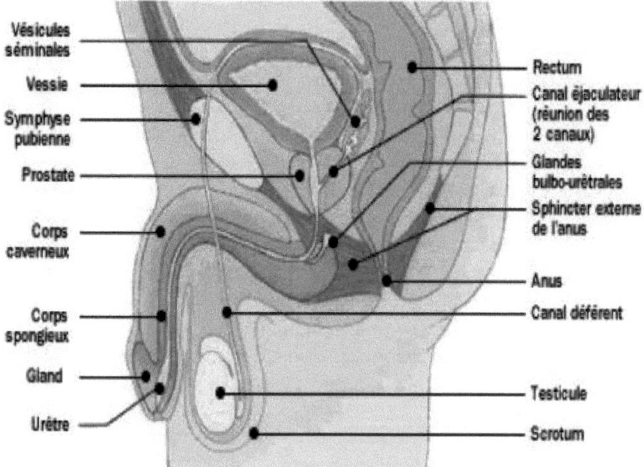

Figure 2: Anatomy of the male genitourinary organs (Profile)
https://microbiologiemedicale.fr/anatomie-physiologie-appareil-genital-masculin/

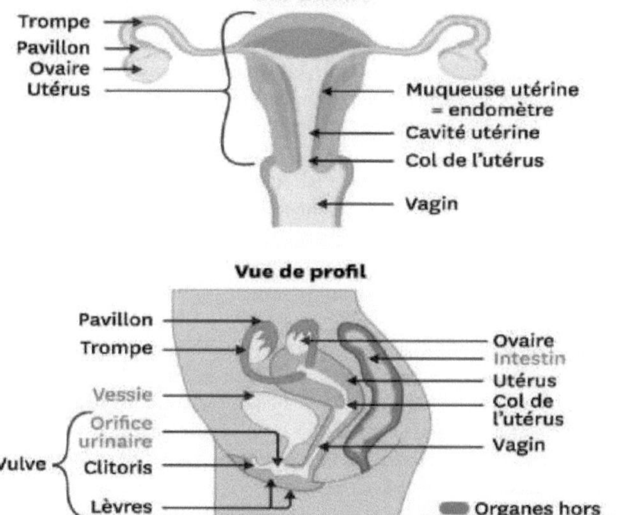

Figure 3: Anatomy of the female genitalia (face and profile) https://microbiologiemedicale.fr/anatomie-physiologie-appareil-genital-feminin

References

1. Vigue-Marin. Atlas of human anatomy. Editions Desiris 2004
2. Netter FH. Altas d'anatomie humaine 5e edition Elsevier Masson 2011
3. Siboulet A, Coulaud JB. Sexually transmitted diseases. Abreges. 2ed Ed Masson 1991

II. Genital discharge

Table 3: Main germs that can colonise the genital mucosa and cause genital discharge [1].

First group	Aerobic saprophytic bacteria: lactobacillus, diphteroid, white and gold staphylococci, enterococci, streptococci and hemolytic bacteria, Gardenerella vaginalis Anaerobic saprophytic bacteria : Propionibacterium species, Actinomyces species, peptostreptococci, Veilonella parvula, bacteroides
Second group	Bacteria: Streptococcus B, Haemophilus influenzae, *Haemophilus parainfluenzae,* Gram-negative bacilli, *Fusobacterium species. Candida albicans, C.glabratta* Mycoplasmas: *Ureaplasma urealyticum, Mycoplasma hominis, Mycoplasma genitalium*
Third group	*Neisseria gonorrhoeae, Chlamydia trachomatis, Trichomonas Vaginalis*

[1] Chambers CVET al. Microflora of urethra in adolescent boys: relationship to sexual activity and gonococcal urethritis. J Pediatr 1987; 110 :314-21

Neisseria gonorrhoeae **infections**

1. Causal agent

Neisseria are "coffee-bean" shaped negative cocci associated with diplococci. They are strict aerobic bacteria with respiratory metabolism only. Isolation of Neisseria requires culture media rich in CO2. Neisseria *gonorrhoeae* (NG) is a strictly human parasite, found in the mucous membranes of the genital tract of both men and women [2].

The gonococcus was first observed by Neisser in 1879 in urethral pus, and in 1882 Leistikov and Loeffler produced the first culture on coagulated serum [2]. This is the agent of gonorrhoea, which has been known since antiquity. Indeed, the first description was made by a Chinese emperor in 2637 BC. Gonococcal disease was identified by Ricord in 1830 [3]. It is still called gonorrhoea or gonococcal gonorrhoea or "hot piss" because of the painful symptoms it causes in acute urethral forms. It is caused by *Neisseria gonorrhoeae*. Symptoms vary considerably according to sex.

2. Symptoms

In men

NG develops rapidly in the genital tract. The incubation period varies between 2 and 10 days (average 6 days).

In the common ийиё form, gonococcal disease in men manifests itself as more or less extensive, purulent, sometimes whitish or yellowish, urethral discharge. Urine discharges are painful ("the patient pees razor blades") [4, 5]. The tip of the urethra (meat) is red and tender. The urine is cloudy with filaments (at this stage, only the first glass of urine is cloudy). There is little or no fever. The patient complains of pollakiuria and dysuria. In some severe forms, the patient may emit a few drops of blood at the end of micturition; in exceptional cases, haemospermia may be observed. The spontaneous evolution is towards loco-regional complications [5].

In sub-acute forms, symptoms are less obvious. There is no clear urethral discharge; at most, the patient observes morning drops, a spot in the pants or sensations of intra-urethral pruritus [4-6]. In some cases, it may be isolated pyuria. These sulcus or chronic forms may be relapses or recurrences that are neglected or poorly treated. Urethritis manifests itself as a whitish, thinner drop seen in the morning on waking. These are generally small foci created by the gonococcus and maintained by common germs. These sulcus and chronic forms are the source of complications.

Complications: Uncommon in men, these complications are observed in the course of urethritis that has been treated late or neglected [7]. They involve the various glandular formations attached to the anterior and posterior urethra, as well as the epididymo-deferential apparatus.

- Involvement of the epididymitis and vas deferens is marked by increasing spontaneous pain at the level of a bursa, radiating along the cords, with or without a thermal hook (39 and 40°C). Sometimes the epididymis increases in volume and covers the testicle. The pain may go up the spermatic cord and palpation of the epididymis is particularly painful in the tail area. Palpation often reveals a painful epididymo-testicular block that makes walking and standing more or less impossible. Isolated orchitis is rarely seen in gonococcal disease. Treatment must be early and very prolonged, as there is a high risk of a scarring nucleus interrupting the sperm excretory pathway. Bilateral involvement (in one or more stages) can lead to permanent male sterility. A bilateral epididymal nucleus is found in 30% of sterile men [8-10].
- Prostatitis: Prolonged involvement, with pain in the perineum, a painful gene when passing urine and a fever of 38-39°C. A rectal examination reveals a prostate that is more or less enlarged. In severe cases, acute prostatitis can lead to prostatic abscess with pain on discharge, tenesmus, acute urine retention, sometimes due to bladder spasm, and fistulisation in the posterior ureter or the skin of the perineum. Antibiotic treatment becomes difficult. Few drugs concentrate sufficiently in the prostate, and prolonged treatment (6 weeks to 3 months) is needed to completely cure acute prostatitis.
- Involvement of the small glands around the urethra (Littre's gland: littritis; Cowper's gland: cowperitis; Tyson's gland: tysonitis) is the cause of recurrence and chronic infection.
- Extension of the infection to the ejaculatory ducts and semen vesicles typically causes imperious micturition, terminal hematuria, hemospermia, and pain on erection and ejaculation.
- Involvement of the urethral submucosa results in several peri-urethral abscesses (and may lead to a large urethral abscess). Physical examination reveals infiltration of the corpus spongiosum, leading to painful erections.
- Urethral stricture is a late complication that is currently rare. It is characterised by urethral stenosis manifested by difficult micturition throughout its duration; the strength of the urinary stream is altered (the subject "pisses on his feet"). Urethral stricture usually occurs between 6 months and 2 years after neglected or inadequately treated gonococcal urethritis and may lead to male infertility [11].

In women

Gonococcal disease in women is generally silent, unlike in men (in 8 out of 10 cases, it is asymptomatic or only slightly symptomatic) [12-15]. It is almost always discovered by chance during a check-up for vaginal discharge or during screening after the male partner's gonococcal infection has been discovered.

Clinically it can be :

- discrete urethritis manifested by dysuria, a sensation of heat or burning on urination; the meat is generally normal. Gynaecological examination may reveal a drop of greenish-white pus in the urethra (expression of the urethra on the pubic symphysis);
- cervicitis manifested by leucorrhoea which the patient considers to be commonplace, especially in the case of associated trichomoniasis. This cervicitis can take on a variety of forms: erythematous, erosive, redemato-erythematous. In pregnant women, cervicitis is rapidly purulent. Sometimes this cervicitis leads to dyspareunia and lumbopelvic pain. The infection may be reduced to a few translucent cysts embedded in the mucosa around the cervical os;
- salpingitis: gonococcal salpingitis accounts for 20% of cases of salpingitis [15] (in a third to a quarter of cases, *Chlamydia trachomatis is* found at the same time). PID is the most feared complication of gonococcal disease in women. Typically, gonococcal salpingitis develops acutely. Clinical symptoms of pelvic infection generally appear after the first or second menstrual flow following infection. The patient presents with spontaneous uni- or bilateral abdominal-pelvic pain associated with fever and transit disorders (vomiting, constipation). Questioning often reveals the presence of leucorrhoea in the preceding days. Abdominal palpation reveals tenderness or even contracture, and mobilisation of the cervix during vaginal examination reveals pain, as does

palpation of the cul de sac of Douglas during rectal examination.

Complications

Since most female gonococcal disease is asymptomatic, it is a source of complications that often allow retrospective diagnosis [14, 15].

- *Uretro-skenitis*: Skene's glands may be affected. The expression of the urethra on the pubic symphysis brings back a drop of pus.
- *Acute bartholinitis*: This manifests as general signs (fever) and local signs (perineal pain). Examination reveals a warm, red tumour with swelling of one of the large lips. The spontaneous evolution is towards abcessation or fistulisation in the vestibule or towards sulxuguc' or chronic bartholinitis.
- *Annexitis uðuë (salpingitis) or subaigi^s or chronic adnexitis* with uni or bilateral tumefaction. PID is the leading cause of secondary infertility (ectopic pregnancy, sterility) in women in developing countries.
- *Peritonitis*: abdominal pain and tenderness, transit problems and general signs.
- *Perihepatitis or Fitz Hugh and Curtis syndrome*: This is seen mainly in female sex workers who are more frequently infected. It manifests as moderate abdominal pain in the right hypochondrium, digestive problems such as nausea, asthenia and a moderate deterioration in general condition. Laparoscopy shows a depolished peritoneum with multiple fiddle-string adhesions (this syndrome can also be seen in *Chlamydia trachomatis* infection).

In both sexes

Pharyngeal gonococcal disease: This is relatively common because of genital-oral sexual practices. It is found in 3 to 7% of heterosexual men and 12 to 16% of women, and in over 30% of homosexual men [17, 18]. Clinically, pharyngeal gonococcal disease is asymptomatic in over 85% of cases [16]. Patients complain of a moderate sore throat, with mild redness of the tonsils and pharyngeal mucosa on examination, suggestive of common erythematous angina. More rarely, a purulent exudate may be seen on the tonsils. There are no general signs. Pharyngeal gonococcal disease can serve as a gateway for septicemic dissemination of gonococcus, making it potentially serious. In addition, many patients, particularly MSM, may have multiple sites of infection (urethral, pharyngeal and anorectal). Hence the importance in this group of taking a pharyngeal sample in the event of urethritis.

Anorectal gonorrhoea: This accounts for at least 8-10% of female gonorrhoea and 4-6% of male gonorrhoea. It is more common in MSM [19]. Direct inoculation is the usual route of infection following anal intercourse: 40% of women with anorectal gonococcal disease have had anal intercourse [18]. Self-infection is exceptional in men (from urethritis, from the opening of a prostatic abscess in the rectum, from a Cowper's gland), and more frequent in women (spread from the vicinity via vaginal secretions). Clinically, the acute form manifests as anorectitis (rare). The incubation period, generally lasting 2 to 5 days, is marked by sensations of painful anorectal cooking, burning, heaviness and purulent secretions. The pain is exacerbated by prolonged sitting, walking and defecation, and is accompanied by tenesmus and false urgency, leading to the emission of purulent, usually greenish-yellow secretions. The anal canal is hypercongestive, and the hypertrophic radial folds are covered with purulent streaks which may mask very painful pseudo-fissure ulcerations. In the sulxuguc' form, which is mainly expressed endoscopically, functional problems are generally very discreet. Occasionally, the patient will report mild pruritus, a feeling of anal discomfort, slight oozing with or without blood, and rarely, severe pain on defecation (fissure-like). The most typical appearance is the presence of pus on an apparently healthy mucosa: the anal mucosa is diffusely red, and the rectum is more or less inflamed, suggesting "hemorrhoidal congestion".

In MSM, gonococcal infection of the partner should lead to proctological examination and rectal sampling of sexual partners [19, 20]. Anorectal gonococcal disease is rarely complicated. Abscesses and fistulisations may be observed, which may constitute a potential focus for septic

dissemination [19].
Ocular gonorrhoea: As a result of the widespread prophylactic use of antibiotics, the number of cases of ocular localization has fallen considerably, and they have generally lost their formidable severity. Suppurative conjunctivitis in newborns (contaminated by an infected mother during passage through the genital tract) appears on the 3rd day after birth (the rate of contamination from infected mothers is over 40%) [21, 22]. The newborn's face is quickly deformed by the reddening of the eyelids, which are glued together by purulent, greenish-yellow secretions. Conjunctivitis is red, congestive and haemorrhagic. In the absence of treatment, corneal complications are frequent (ulceration, perforation, cecitis); ophthalmia, which includes conjunctivitis, keratitis, ulceration and corneal perforation, is rarer.

Extra-urogenital and systemic manifestations

Septicemia. This complication is rare nowadays because of the wide access to care and antibiotic therapy. The septicemic spread of gonococcal disease is responsible for a variety of extra-genital localisations. In women, gonococcal dissemination is favoured by pregnancy and menstruation. Gonococcal septicaemia has been reported in immunocompromised patients, with skin, joint and fever manifestations [23, 24]. Rarely, severe sepsis with thrombophlebitis has been reported.

Joint complications. Since the widespread use of antibiotics, gonococcal arthritis has become extremely rare. Joint manifestations are characterised by their clinical polymorphism: there may be polyarthritis affecting mainly the wrists, ankles, knees, fingers, elbows and shoulders, or tenosynovitis [23]. However, in around half of cases, this polyarthritis will be accompanied by a skin rash (macular papules, eruption of bullous vesicles occurring at the extremities or in the vicinity of the affected joints).

Digestive disease: This is perihepatitis or Fitz-Hugh-Curtis syndrome. This syndrome is described in women in whom NG infection is often asymptomatic and goes unnoticed for a long time. It results from direct diffusion of NG from a genital focus to the subphrenic spaces. The germ travels up the fallopian tubes, then the right parietocolonic gutter to the hepatic region. In humans, perihepatic infection is thought to result from hematogenous diffusion or from travel to the liver via the retroperitoneal lymphatic vessels. Clinically, it is a painful syndrome of the right hypochondrium radiating into the shoulder, accentuated by coughing. This painful syndrome is accompanied by nausea. Palpation reveals a painful contracture of the right hypochondrium. There may be urogenital signs (dysuria, burning, leucorrhoea). The differential diagnosis is acute cholecystitis [14].

Meningitis. In recent years, cases of meningitis have been described among MSM. But the causal agent is *Neisseria meningitidis*, which usually colonises the ENT sphere. It is also found in urethritis in this population group, where epidemics have been reported in the United States [24].

3. Diagnosis

Positive diagnosis.

Gonococcal disease is based on the notion of contaminating sexual intercourse, the incubation period and the characteristics of the discharge. However, the diversity of clinical pictures makes diagnosis difficult, and only paraclinical examinations confirm the diagnosis by isolating the germ. Direct examination is easily performed using a smear of the discharge spread on a slide and stained with methylene blue or Gram. The sensitivity of this test compared with culture is excellent, close to 100% [8]. A near-certainty of gonococcal infection is provided by the discovery of extra- and especially intracellular Gram-negative diplococci. The mere presence of extracellular diplococci only provides a presumptive element (it may be a saprophytic Neisseria). Exceptionally, the discovery of intra- and extra-cellular diplococci indicates the presence of meningococcus. Culture on chocolate gelose (Thayer-Martin medium) is the reference test in practice, confirming the diagnosis in 24 to 48 hours. It is used to test for beta-lactamase and to perform an antibiotic susceptibility test. It is carried out on the discharge if there is one, by anourethral swab if there is no discharge, or on the first urine stream (although the latter technique is less sensitive).

Rapid diagnosis is based on nucleic acid amplification tests (NAATs): most of these tests are duplex *N. gonorrhoeae/C. trachomatis* [3, 8, 25]. In asymptomatic subjects, tests are performed on the first urine stream. In the event of a positive test, a culture should be taken in order to perform an antibiotic susceptibility test. In complications where there is no longer any discharge, immunological techniques (indirect immunofluorescence) can be of great help in making an etiological diagnosis. In current practice, two serological reactions are taken into consideration: indirect immunofluorescence and the hemagglutination reaction are suggestive of gonococcal infection.

Differential diagnosis

In humans. The acute form does not generally pose any diagnostic problems. In sulcus or chronic forms, the diagnosis should be discussed with non-gonococcal urethritis [2]. (Chlamydia, trichomoniasis, candidiasis, mycoplasma infection). Urethritis of mixed etiology is relatively common. In all cases, bacteriological samples should be taken to establish the uniqueness of the etiology of urethritis and to rule out other causes. In the event of complications, particularly epididymitis, other possible causes should be discussed: a transparent cyst of the epididymis; orchiepididymitis associated with influenza or mumps; tuberculous epididymitis (nuclei on the head and tail); colibacillary, staphylococcal, mycoplasma or chlamydial epididymitis.

In women. Vulvovaginitis due to candida or trichomonas must be ruled out. These are very noisy, unlike gonococcus, which is paucisymptomatic. Differential diagnosis with chlamydiosis is more difficult, and only paraclinical examinations can clarify the etiology. PID poses the problem of its multiple etiologies (sexually transmitted and/or non-sexually transmitted germs).

4. Treatment

The aim is to rapidly destroy the gonococcus in order to avoid complications and break the chains of contamination as quickly as possible.

Many antibiotics can be used to treat gonococcal disease. The sensitivity of gonococcus to antibiotics is constantly changing and varies from one country to another, and within the same country from one place to another. Therapeutic recommendations therefore vary in time and space. They must be constantly updated because of the resistance of *N. gonorrhoeae* to antibiotics (beta lactamase-producing strains) [26].

The antibiotics currently active in most countries are the subject of consensus recommendations for the treatment of gonococcal disease.

Ceftriaxone: a single intramuscular injection of 500 mg. This third-generation cephalosporin is effective and remains the first-line treatment [8, 26]. It is also the antibiotic of choice in cases of associated pharyngeal gonorrhoea. Its tolerance is excellent. The only contraindications are anticoagulant therapy and allergy to penicillin. It should be emphasised that third-generation oral cephalosporins are not recommended because of their poorer bioavailability and the frequency of digestive problems, making them less effective and exposing *N. gonorrhoeae to* the acquisition of resistance.

Azithromycin is effective with high doses of around 2g. The side-effects are mainly digestive problems. In practice, one of the major advantages of this antibiotic is that it is also effective against *Chlamydia trachomatis* at a single dose, making it possible to treat the two most common and most morbid infections, NG and CT [26]. However, resistance has already been reported with this compound.

Gentamycin 240 mg intramuscularly in a single dose may be proposed in specific situations of contraindication or in combination [50, 51].

Zoliflodacin is the new antibiotic with a single dose efficacy of over 95% [27].

References

1. Chambers CV, Strafer Man Adjer H et al. Microflora of urethra in adolescent boys: relationship to sexual activity and gonococcal urethritis. J Pediatr 1987 ; 110 :314-21

2. Chaine B, Janier M. Uretrites. EMC (Elsevier Masson SAS, Paris). Dermatology 98-440- A-10, 2010

3. Gerhardt P, Dupin N, Janier M et al. Male urethritis. Ann Dermatol Venereol 2016; 143: 752-55

4. Pitche P. Urethritis. EMC -Dermatology 2022 (2) [article 98-440- A-10].

5. Janier M, Lassau F, Cassin I et al. Male urethritis with and without discharge: clinical and microbiological study. Sex Transm Dis 1995; 22: 244-252

6. Rowley J, Vander-hoom S, Korenromp E et al. Chlamydia, gonorrheae, trichomiasis and syphilis. Global prevalence and incidence estimates. Bull Word health Organ 2019; 97: 548562

7. Newman L.M, Moran JS, Workowski KA. Up date on the management of gonorrhea in a adults in the United States. Clin Infect Dis 2007; 44(Suppl 3) : S84-101.

8. Centers for Diseases Control and Prevention. Sexually transmitted infections treatement. Guidelines 2021. MMR 2021; 70: 30-59

9. Trojian TH, Timothy S Lishnak TS et al. Epididymitis and orchitis: an overview. Am Fam Physician 2009;79 :583-7.

10. Hamill MM, Annet Onzia A, Wang TH et al.High burden of untreated syphilis, drug resistant *Neisseria gonorrhoeae*, and other sexually transmitted infections in men with urethral discharge syndrome in Kampala, Uganda. BMC Infect Dis 2022 7; 22:440. doi: 10.1186/s12879-022-07431-1.

11. Unemo M, Seifert HS, Hook EW 3rd et al. Gonorrhoea. Nat Rev Dis Primers 2019; 5(1): 79. doi: 10.1038/s41572-019-0128-6.

12. Kassa ZK, Hussen S, Nebiha Hadra Net al. Prevalence of *Neisseria gonorrhoeae* infection among women of reproductive age in sub-Saharan Africa: a systematic review and metaanalysis. Eur J Contracept Reprod Health Care 2020; 25: 365-371.

13. Kularatne RS, Nil R, Rowley J et al. Adult gonorrhea, chlamydia and syphilis prevalence, incidence and syndromic case reporting in South Africa. PloS One 2018; 13 (10) e205863 Epub 2018 Oct 5

14. Rostami MN, Rashidi BH, Habibi A et al. Genital infections and reproductive complications associated with Trichomonas vaginalis, Neisseria gonorrhoeae, and Streptococcus agalactiae in women of Qom, central Iran. Int J Reprod Biomed. 2017; 15: 357366.

15. Dubbink JH, Verweij SP, Helen E Struthers HE et al. Genital *Chlamydia trachomatis* and *Neisseria gonorrhoeae* infections among women in sub-Saharan Africa: A structured review Int J STD AIDS 2018;29:806-824.

16. Blank S, Doskalakis DC. *Nesseiria gonorrhoeae*. Rising infection rates. Dwinding treatement options. N Engl J Med 2018; 379: 1795-97

17. Philip A, Chan PA, Robinette A et al. Extragenital Infections Caused by *Chlamydia trachomatis* and *Neisseria gonorrhoeae:* A Review of the Literature. Infect Dis Obstet Gynecol 2016;16:575-83.

18. Adamson PC, Bhatia R, Tran KD et al. Prevalence, Anatomic Distribution, and Correlates of *Chlamydia trachomatis* and *Neisseria gonorrhoeae* Infections Among a Cohort of Men Who Have Sex With Men in Hanoi, Vietnam. Sex Transm Dis 2022;49:504-510.

19. Ramadhani HO, Liu H, Nowak RG et al. Sexual partner characteristics and incident rectal *Neisseria gonorrhoeae* and *Chlamydia trachomatis* infections among gay men and other men who have sex with men (MSM): a prospective cohort in Abuja and Lagos, Nigeria Sex Transm Infect 2017;93:348-355.

20. Hascoet JL, Dahoun M, Cohen M et al. Clinical diagnostic and therapeutic aspects of 221 consecutive anorectal *Chlamydia trachomatis* and *Neisseria gonorrhoeae* sexually transmitted infections among men who have sex with men. Int J Infect Dis 2018 ;71:9-13.

21. Vaezzadeh K, A, Nayereh As'adi N et al. Global prevalence of *Neisseria gonorrhoeae* infection in pregnant women: a systematic review and meta-analysis. Clin Microbiol Infect 2023

;29:22-31.
22. Mehlen M, Saunier V, de Barbeyrac B et al. Keep an eye on *Neisseria gonorrhoeae.* Clin Microbiol Infect. 2020;26:1183-1184.
23. Russ-Friedman C, Coates K, Torab M et al. *Neisseria gonorrhoeae* septic arthritis with contiguous infection consistent with acute osteomyelitis. Sex Transm Dis 2020; 47:e36-e38.
24. 25 MaatoukI.Neisseria meningitidis urethritis: synthesis of published data Int J Dermatol2018;57(8):e48-e49. doi: 10.1111/ijd.14060. Epub 2018 May 24.
25. Unemo M, Ross JDC, Serwin AB et al. 2020 European guideline for the diagnosis and treatment of gonorrhea in adults. Int J STD AIDS 2020;29 :956462420949126. doi :10.1177/0956462420949126.
26. Barbee LA Kerani RP, Dombrowski JC et al. A retrospective comparative study of 2-drug oral and intramuscular cephalosporin treatment regimens for pharyngeal gonorrhea. Clin Infect Dis 2013;56:1539-45.
27. Taylor SN, Marrazzo J, Bateiger BE et al. Single-dose zoliflodacin (ETX0914) for treatement of urogenital gonorrhea. New Engl J Med 2018; 379: 1835-45

Chlamydia trachomatis **infection**

1. Causal agent

In 1906, Haelberstaeder and Von Prowazk discovered inclusions in the conjunctival smears of trichomatous organisms [1]. In 1964, Moulder showed that these inclusions were intracellular developing bacteria [1]. The genus Chlamydia belongs to the Chlamydiaceae family and comprises three species*: C. trachomatis, C. psittaci and C. pneumoniae* [2]. Humans are the exclusive host of *C. trachomatis.* Serovars A, B and C are responsible for trachoma and are transmitted indirectly by dirty hands, objects and flies; serovars D to K are responsible for genitourinary, ocular and pulmonary infections; serovars L1, L2 and L3 are responsible for lymphogranulomatosis venereum [1, 3].
The role of *Chlamydia trachomatis* in the occurrence of 1ST is a recent finding. We now know that in Europe and North America, *Chlamydia trachomatis is* found in 60% of men with non-gonococcal urethritis [3, 4]. Infection is found in 80% of female partners of men with gonorrhoea, without them having the slightest symptoms or a non-evocative leucorrhoea. *Chlamydia trachomatis* is responsible for 40-60% of cases of PID. The high frequency of CT infections in both sexes favours its spread in the sexually active population.

2. Symptomatology

In men

The incubation period is often difficult to specify, ranging from 4 to 15 days (extreme 4 days to 30 days) or even a few months, and is usually impossible to define [4, 5]. This incubation period is contagious and plays an important epidemiological role in the spread of the infection. In more than half of cases, the infection is asymptomatic. When it is symptomatic, it is generally sulxuguc' urethritis [5-7]. It manifests as a light, clear, intermittent discharge, often in the morning, which is almost always painless. Functional signs are more or less discreet, with some burning, mild pruritus or a simple isolated morning drop. In 5-10% of cases, the clinical picture is of acute urethritis with purulent discharge and painful micturition, which is difficult to distinguish from gonococcal urethritis [6].
Given that most of them are paucisymptomatic or asymptomatic, there are a few complications.
Epididymitis or orchiepididymitis occurs in young subjects (50-70% of causes of acute orchiepididymitis) [7, 8] and may be uni or bilateral. Acute or chronic prostatitis accounts for the vast majority of abnormalities, and transrectal ultrasound is a useful diagnostic tool. Cowperitis is exceptional. Proctitis may occur in cases of ano-genital intercourse. Urethritis caused by C. trachomatis may be responsible for Fiessinger-Leroy-Reiter syndrome [9, 10]. This is a reactive arthritis that occurs after urethritis, most often in young men, and combines: bilateral

conjunctivitis, joint signs (acute or subacute asymmetric polyarthritis affecting mainly the large joints of the lower limbs, talalgia or tendonitis) and mucocutaneous signs (circinate balanitis, psoriasiform lesions). Apart from urethritis, C. trachomatis can be isolated from pharyngeal (with or without pharyngitis) and anorectal swabs, particularly in MSM (men who have sex with men) [11, 12].

In women. The clinical manifestations are generally fairly trivial and most often asymptomatic, but the risk of infection of the upper tract, which can lead to salpingitis, makes them particularly serious [4, 6]. The incubation period is impossible to specify in more than 75% of cases; it is estimated at between 8 and 15 days (extreme 4 to 30 days).

Symptomatic forms are characterised by isolated leucorrhoea with no other subjective manifestations. Speculum examination reveals signs of cervical inflammation, either isolated inflammation of the ectocervix or endocervix, or erosive cervicitis. In other cases, there is subacute vulvovaginitis, with more or less abundant leucorrhoea, pruritus or vulvovaginal burning and sometimes dyspareunia, which may resemble the clinical picture of acute female gonococcal disease [6]. In some cases, there are no objective or subjective functional signs, and only speculum examination reveals exo or endocervicitis.

In women, Chlamydia trachomatis infection is particularly morbid, causing multiple complications that often lead to sterility (the leading cause of secondary sterility in southern countries). Pelviperitonitis and perihepatitis (FitzHugh-Curtis syndrome) are also possible. PID occurs in young women and is the most serious complication. It may be acute salpingitis with pelvic pain, often unilateral, which may be associated with metrorrhagia and fever. PID is often silent and is the cause of infertility and tubal sterility in women [13-15].

In both sexes.

Conjunctivitis. Conjunctivitis can also occur in adults: it may be isolated or associated with other sites (urethritis or Fiessinger Leroy Reiter syndrome). It is often unilateral and spontaneously regresses in the majority of cases [10].

Sphere-buccopharyngeal involvement. Pharyngeal involvement is common in MSM and heterosexual men and women who have oral sex. Clinically, the signs are those of pharyngitis, but in the majority of cases, the disease is asymptomatic and is discovered during screening [16]. Stomatitis of the palate or inner cheeks has also been described, characterised by smooth, superficial, erythematous macular lesions. Glossitis appears in the form of an oval plaque, sometimes with the appearance of a geographical map, which may give rise to discussion of several etiologies when it is isolated [14].

Anal involvement. It manifests itself in the form of seropurulent secretions. This site is common in MSM [3].

Joint involvement. This is often reported as part of Fiessinger Leroy Reiter syndrome, but may also be isolated [9]. Clinical symptoms include arthralgia or low back pain, often transient. The majority of cases involve the knees, sacroiliac joints, tibio-tarsal joints and joints of the big toe (or feet). Talalgia is fairly suggestive in sexually active adults (with no other obvious etiology). The synovial fluid is inflammatory, with inclusions in the synovial cells.

Fiessinger-Leroy-Reiter syndrome. This is the classic ureteroconjunctivosynovial syndrome [9]. Fiessinger-Leroy-Reiter syndrome is characterised by the triad of oligoarthritis affecting the large joints of the lower limbs, urethritis and conjunctivitis. However, incomplete forms of reactive arthritis are common and may take the form of monoarthritis or naked oligoarthritis. Atypical forms have also been described, with various cutaneous and mucosal manifestations: erythematosquamous or pustular macules; keratotic lesions with suggestive involvement of the soles of the feet and hands [10]. The course of reactive arthritis is marked by the risk of relapse in 20% to 50% of patients [10]. The pathogenesis of the syndrome is still unclear, and is thought to be characterised by the amplification of the inflammatory response to contact with the triggering bacteria [17]. The exact role of the HLA-B27 molecule is still not fully understood. Several studies have shown the presence and persistence of bacterial antigens within the affected joints (in fact, apart from CT, other germs are involved in the onset of Reiter's syndrome), raising the question of the relevance of antibiotic treatment [9]. While antibiotic treatment is essential for urogenital infections with *Chlamydia trachomatis,* as it prevents or reduces the occurrence of reactive arthritis when given early, this is not the case for post-enteritis arthritis [9].

Children and infants

In infants and small children, *Chlamydia trachomatis* causes pneumopathy or interstitial pneumonia (perinatal vaginal contamination and spread to the respiratory tract) and conjunctivitis neonatorum or ophthalmia neonatorum [17]. *Chlamydia trachomatis* is responsible for at least 30% of neonatal conjunctivitis [17, 18]. This is a mucopurulent conjunctivitis, contracted when the foetus passes through the mother's genital tract at the time of delivery. CT pneumonia is clinically unremarkable, and may be isolated or associated with conjunctivitis, particularly in neonates or young infants, thus confirming the role of maternal transmission.

3. Diagnosis

Positive diagnosis of *C. trachomatis* genital chlamydia is based on paraclinical examinations [5, 16, 19-21]. The reference test for the diagnosis of *C. trachomatis* infection is culture on HeLa 229 or MacCoy cells. It is 100% specific in all cases. However, this test takes a long time (3 to 7 days), is difficult and expensive, is reserved for specialist laboratories and requires an endo-urethral sample (3 to 4 centimetres) or a sample taken from the endocervix, by scraping the epithelium with a swab [5]. As urine is toxic for cultures, cultures cannot be taken from the first urine stream. As *C. trachomatis is* an obligate intra-cellular bacterium, present in epithelial cells, it is not visible on a simple urethral smear. The only rapid tests available are direct slide immunofluorescence (30 to 40 minutes) or enzyme-linked immunosorbent assays (3 to 4 hours), which are around 90% specific but only 70 to 80% sensitive. They are easy to perform but require an endo-urethral sample. The sensitivity of these tests on the first urine jet in men is still low (25-80%).

C. trachomatis genomic amplification reactions (PCR) are highly sensitive, slightly better than culture. Their great advantage is that they can be performed on the first urine stream [20, 21]. Rapid diagnosis is based on nucleic acid amplification tests (NAATs). Serodiagnosis of *C. trachomatis is of* no value in the diagnosis of uncomplicated genital chlamydial infections. However, given the prevalence and morbidity of chlamydia infection in under-resourced developing countries, serodiagnosis provides strong presumptive diagnostic evidence. In certain complicated forms (pulmonary involvement, salpingitis, epididymitis), antibody measurement (increase in antibodies between two serums) enables the diagnosis to be made and, in some cases, excess treatment to be given. Several techniques (complement fixation reaction, micro-immunofluorescence technique: ELISA type) are used [21]. However, only the Westernblot or immuno-transfer technique can distinguish the nature of the antibodies involved in the immune reaction. This technique makes it possible to judge the profile of the antibodies and their nature, and to relate them to an evolving stage of the disease.

The differential diagnosis is essentially gonococcal urethritis in men and other causes of cervicitis in women [22]. Conjunctivitis and Reiter's syndrome should be discussed for their other etiologies with a view to appropriate treatment.

4. Treatment

Three criteria govern the choice of treatment for urethro-genital infections with *Chlamydia trachomatis: in vitro* bacteriological efficacy; duration of treatment sufficient to eliminate any complications; possibility of epidemiological treatment of sexual partners [7, 23-25].

The antibiotics effective in vitro against *C. trachomatis* are cyclins and macrolides. The recommended treatment regimens are :

- doxycycline 200 mg once-daily: improved therapeutic adherence. The adverse effects of cyclins consist mainly of digestive problems, but also toxidermia and photosensitisation. In uncomplicated genital infections *caused by C. trachomatis,* a 7-day course of treatment is just as effective as a longer course. A higher dosage does not bring any substantial benefit. Therapeutic failures are due to recontamination, poor digestive absorption, possibly poor diffusion of the antibiotics, and above all poor compliance. Cyclins are contraindicated in pregnant women.

- azithromycin: a single oral dose of 1g. This new macrolide (azalide) has a very long half-life (72 hours) and high tissue and cell diffusion, and is as effective in a single dose as 7 days of doxycycline. Tolerance is excellent. Despite its high cost. This type of treatment represents a real revolution in the management of *C. trachomatis* infections.

For conjunctivitis in newborns, erythromycin 50 mg/kg/d (taken four times a day) for 14 days or azithromycin 20 mg/kg/d once a day for 3 days is suggested.

Azithromycin and erythromycin are indicated for use in pregnant and breastfeeding women and in children.

References

1. Avril JL, Dabernat H, Denis F et al. Bacteriologie clinique, 2edition. Ellipses 1992

2. Freney J, Riegel P. Bacteriologie clinique 3[e] edition ESKA 2018

3. Robinso TD. The discovery of *Chlamydia trachomatis*. Sex Transm Infect 2017;93:10. doi: 10.1136/sextrans-2016-053011.

4. Rowley J, Vander-hoom S, Korenromp E et al. Chlamydia, gonorrheae, trichomiasis and syphilis. Global prevalence and incidence estimates. Bull Word health Organ 2019; 97: 548562

3. Kato Y, Kawaguchi S, Shigehara K et al. Prevalence of N. gonorrhoeae, C. trachomatis, M. genitalium, M. hominis and Ureaplasma spp in the anus and urine among Japanese HIV-infected men who have sex with men. J Infect Chemother 2019 Dec 24. Pi: S1314-1341- 321X(19)30376-9.doi 10.1016/j.jiac.2019.12.007.

4. Blair CS, Garner OB, Pedone B et al. Factors associated with repeat rectal Neisseria gonorrhoeae and Chlamydia trachomatis screening following inconclusive nucleic acid amplification testing: potential missed opportunity for screening. PloS One, 2019 Dec 12;14:e0226413.doi 10.1371/journal.pone.0226413. eCollection 2019.

5. Dupin N, Janier M, Bousacart F et al. *Chlamydia trachomatis*. Ann Dermatol Venereol 2016; 143: 713-15

6. Touati A, Vernay-Vaisse C, Janier M et al. People With Genital *Chlamydia trachomatis* Infection in France in 2013. Sex Transm Dis 2016;43:374-6.

7. Centers for Diseases Control and Prevention. Sexually transmitted infections treatement. Guidelines 2021. MMR 2021; 70: 30-59

8. Trei JS, Carres LC, Gould PL. Reproductive tract complications associated Chlamydia trachomatis infections in US Air Force males whithin 4 years testing. Sex Transm Dis 2008; 35: 827-33

9. Gerard HC, Branigan PJ, Schumacher Jr HR et al. Synovial Chlamydia trachomatis in patients with reactive arthritis/Reiter's syndrome are viable but show aberrant gene expression. J Rheumatol 1998;25:734-42.

1.1. Bojovic J, Strelic N, Pavlica L. Reiter's syndrome disease of young men: analysis of 312 patients. Med Pregl 2014;67:222-30.

11. O'Connell CM, Ferone ME. *Chlamydia trachomatis* Genital Infections. Microb Cell 2016 ;3:390-403

12. Otieno F, Ngety G, Okall D et al. Incidence gonorrhoea and chlamydia among a prospective cohort of men who have sex with men in Kisumun Kenya. Sex Transm Infect 2020 Jan 23. Pii: sextrans-2019-054166. doi: 10.136/sextrans-2019-05416.

13. Lopez-Hudardo M, Velazco-Fernandez M et al. Molecular detection of Chlamydia trachomatis and sem quality of sexual partners of infertile women. Andrologia 2018; 50 (1) doi. 10.1111/and.12812.

14. Hoenderboom BM, van Benthen BHB, van Berger JE et al. Relation between *Chlamydia trachomatis* infections and pelvic disease, ectopic pregnancy and tubual factor infertility in

women.
Dutch cohort of women previously tested for Chlamydia in a chlamydia screen trial. Sex Transm Infect 2019; 95:300-3006
15. Kularatne RS, Nil R, Rowley J et al. Adult gonorrhea, chlamydia and syphilis prevalence, incidence and syndromic case reporting in South Africa. PloS One 2018; 13: e205863
16. Johnson RE, Green TA, Schachter J et al. Evaluation of nucleic amplification tests as reference tests for Chlamydia trachomatis infections in asymptomatic men. J Clin Microbiol 2000; 38: 4382-86
17. Vodstrcil LA, McIver R, Huston WM et al. The Epidemiology of *Chlamydia trachomatis* organism load during genital infection: A Systematic Review. J Infect Dis. 2015;211:1628-45.
18. Leung AKC, Hon KL, Wong AHC, et al. Bacterial conjunctivitis in Ccildhood: Etiology, licnical manifestations, diagnosis, and management. Recent Pat Inflamm Allergy Drug Discov 2018;12:120-127
19. Black CM. Current methods of laboratory diagnosis of *Chlamydia trachomatis* infections Clin Microbiol Rev 1997;10:160-84.
20. Johnson RE, Green TA, Schachter J et al. Evaluation of nucleic amplification tests as reference tests for *Chlamydia trachomatis* infections in asymptomatic men. J Clin Microbiol 2000; 38: 4382-86
21. Lopez-Hudardo M, Velazco-Fernandez M, Pedrate-Sanchez MJE et al. Molecular detection of *Chlamydia trachomatis* and semen quality of sexual partners of infertile women. Andrologia 2018; 50: doi. 10.1111/and.12812. Epud 2017.
22. Pitche P. Wetrites. EMC -Dermatology 2022 (2) [article 98-440- A-10].
23. Dukers-Muijrers NHTM, Wolffs PFG, De Vries H et al. Treatment Effectiveness of Azithromycin and Doxycycline in Uncomplicated Rectal and Vaginal Chlamydia trachomatis Infections in Women: A Multicenter Observational Study (FemCure). Clin Infect Dis 2019;69:1946-1954.
24. Paez-Carro C, Alzate JP, Gonzalez LM et al. Antibiotic for treating urogenital *Chlamydia trachomatis* infections in men and non-pregnant women. Cochrane Database Syst Rev. 2019 Jan 25;1(1):CD010871. doi: 10.1002/14651858.CD010871
25. Lanjouw E, Ouburg S, de Vries HJ et al. 2015 European guideline on the management of Chlamydia trachomatis infections. Int J STD AIDS. 2016;27:333-48

Mycoplasma infections

1. Causal agent

Mycoplasmas are the smallest known form of autonomous life. They are eubacteria belonging to the tenericutes group (bacteria without a rigid wall). These bacteria are limited only by the cytoplasmic membrane [1].

In 1898, Nocard and Roux isolated a new germ in a case of bovid peripneumonia. In 1929, Nowak proposed the name Mycoplasma to group together these wall-less germs [1, 2]. Since 1973, mycoplasmas have been grouped together in a single class, that of the Mollucites in the order Mycoplasmatales and in the genera Mycoplasma; Ureaplsama and Acholeplasma [2]. The species M. *hominis, M. genitalium and U. urealyticum* are normal hosts of the male and female genital tracts and can be implicated in sexually transmitted diseases. However, the pathological role of certain microorganisms such as M. *hominis* in the occurrence of genital discharge remains to be clarified [3].

2. Symptomatology

In men

M. genitalium is responsible for acute urethritis: it is the second most common cause of non-gonococcal urethritis after *Chlamydia trachomatis*, accounting for 20-35% of non-gonococcal urethritis [46]. It is responsible for 40% of recurrent or persistent urethritis [6]. *U. urealyticum* is responsible for subacute urethritis (morning drop with minimal discharge accompanied by a sensation of pruritus around the meat) or recurrent urethritis. In most cases, these are asymptomatic infections or, in rare cases, mixed causes with other germs such as *Chlamydia trachomatis, Neisseria gonorrhoeae* or *Trichomonas vaginalis [5-7]*. Complications are rare and are linked to the persistence of untreated germs, leading to prostatitis or prostato-vesiculitis or even epididymitis [7].

In women

Mycoplasma infections can manifest themselves in three clinical pictures [68]. These may be :

- of vaginosis. *M. hominis* is frequently found in bacterial vaginosis in more than half of cases. It causes abundant, foul-smelling leucorrhoea, sometimes accompanied by cystalgia.
- cervicitis. *M. genitalium* may be responsible for cervicitis alone or in association with other germs, notably CT or NG in the pelvic inflammatory syndrome. MG is associated with 10-30% of cervicitis and may also be associated with an increased risk of abortion and tubal infertility [8].
- salpingitis or endometritis. *U. urealyticum* is found in certain cases of endometritis and salpingitis.

In both sexes. *M. genitalium* is found in 1 to 26% of cases of infectious rectitis in MSM and 3% in women [9].

3. Diagnosis

Positive diagnosis is based on molecular biology with identification of the germ by PCR, particularly for *M. genitalium*. Specific PCR tests or multiplex tests (NAAT) are available [10-11]. Positive diagnosis makes it possible to distinguish between other causes of genital discharge in both men and women.

4. Treatment

Treatment is aimed specifically at *M. genitalium*; as the pathogenicity of *M. hominis* and *U. urealyticum* is not high, it is not recommended to treat them in practice [7, 12-14].

Doxycycline (100mg twice daily for 7 days) followed by azithromycin 500mg daily for 3 days is the first-line treatment in practice (other cyclins are increasingly ineffective against *M. genitalium*) [7]. In the event of resistance to azithromycin, doxycycline 100 mg twice daily for 7 days is suggested. Moxifloxacin 400 mg daily for 10 to 14 days.

References

1. Freney J, Riegel P. Bacteriologie clinique 3e edition ESKA 2018
2. Anagrius C, Lore B, Jensen JS. *Mycoplasma genitalium:* prevalence clinical significance and transmission. Sex Transm Infect 2005; 81 :458-62
3. McGowin CL, Totten PA. The unique microbiology and molecular pathogenesis of *Mycoplasma genitalium*. J Infect Dis. 2017;216(suppl2): S382-S388
4. Dehon PM, Mc Gowin Cl, The immunopathogenesis of *Mycoplasma genitalium* infections in women: a narrative review. Sem Transm Infect 2011 ;87 :107-9
5. Saria M, Kukul E. Classification of nongonococcal urethritis: a review. Int Urol Nephrol 2019; 51: 901-07
6. Bjartling C, Osser S, Person K. The association between *Mycoplasma genitalium* and pelvic inflammatory disease after termination of pregnancy. BJOG 2010; 117: 316-4
7. Centers for Diseases Control and Prevention. Sexually transmitted infections treatement. Guidelines 2021. MMR 2021; **70**: 30-59
8. Pinto-Sander N, Soni S. *Mycoplasma genitalium* infection. BMJ 2019;367:15820.doi 10.1136/bmj.15820
9. Horner PJ, Martin DH. *Mycoplasma genitalium*: Infection in Men. J Infect Dis. 2017;216(suppl2): S396-S405
10. Horner P, Donders G, Cusini M et al. Should we be testing for urogenital *Mycoplasma hominis, Ureaplasma parvum and Ureaplasma urealytica* in men and women. A position statement from the European STI Guidelines Editorial Board. J Eur Acad Dermatol Venereol

2018; 32: 1845-47.
11. Gnanadurai R, Fifer H. *Mycoplasma genitalium: A* Review. Microbiology (Reading). 2020 ;166:21-29
12. Mena LA, Mroczkowski TF, Nsuami M. A randomized comparison of azithromycin and doxycycline for the treatment of *Mycoplasma genitalium-positive* urethritis in men. Clin infect Dis 2009;48:649-54.
13. Martens L, Kuster S, de Vos et al. Macrolide-Resistant Mycoplasma genitalium in Southeastern Region of Netherland, 2014-2017. Emerg Infect Dis 2019;25:1297-1303
14. Hokynar K, Hiltunen-Back E, Mannonen L et al. Prevalence of *Mycoplasma genitalium* and mutations associated with macrolide and fluoroquinolone resistance in Finland. *Int J STD AIDS 2018 ; 29 :904-907.*

Trichomonas vaginalis **infection**

1. Causal agent

It is a eukaryotic flagellate protozoan belonging to the *Trichomonadidae* family. The microorganism was first described in 1836 by Alfred Donne [1]. Of the three known species, only *Trichomonas vaginalis* is pathogenic to humans. *Trichomonas vaginalis* (TV) is 7 to 23 pm long and 5 to 12 pm wide. The cell body is piliform, with a membrane-bound nucleus and a well-developed endoplasmic reticulum. The parasite moves by means of four free anterior flagella implanted in the blepharoplasete and a fifth connected to the cytoplasmic membrane by the undulating membrane [1]. TV is a flagellate, extracellular motile, anaerobic protozoan that is strictly human and exists only in vegetative form; it is almost exclusively sexually transmitted [2, 3].

2. Symptomatology

In women

Trichomoniasis in women results in vulvovaginitis, most often with a sulxiigucv course. The incubation period is often difficult to define [3]. It ranges from 4 days to 4 weeks.

- The acute form is rare (less than 10% of cases). It manifests as hyperalgesic vulvovaginitis with dyspareunia and profuse leucorrhoea. It presents in much the same way as acute gonococcal vulvovaginitis, with urinary problems such as burning of the micturition, pollakiuria, dysuria and cystalgia [3].
- Subacute forms are the most common (60-70% of cases) [3-5]. They are associated with more or less abundant leucorrhoea, usually frothy, airy and sometimes yellowish. Vulvitis and vaginitis may be observed, initially affecting the anterior third of the vagina and then the entire vagina. This inflammation causes superficial dyspareunia at first, then total dyspareunia, which may lead to the cessation of sexual intercourse. The vaginal mucosa shows a dark red spike, and focal cervicitis in "leopard" macules.
- Asymptomatic forms (15-20% of cases) are discovered incidentally following a systematic examination [6].
- Atypical clinical forms have been described. These may include pain of varying intensity or pelvic heaviness, or metrorrhagia ranging from simple bloody streaks in the leucorrhoea to small haemorrhages occurring after intercourse.

Complications of trichomoniasis are exceptional. Skenitis or bartholinitis may be observed. TV may be associated with a risk of prematurity due to early rupture of the membranes and a risk of low birth weight babies [5-7].

In men

Male trichomoniasis usually manifests as subaigucv urethritis, with an incubation period of between 10 and 30 days. Male circumcision reduces the risk of VT infection [3, 6]. Clinically, the symptoms consist of sulxugucosal urethritis with a mucopurulent discharge in the morning, associated with pruritic sensations within the urethra. This classic morning drop often haunts patients, who maintain the secretion by squeezing their meat every morning. Urethritis шдиё is rare and simulates gonococcal urethritis. Asymptomatic forms are the most common (90% of cases) [6]. They are discovered during screening after the diagnosis of infection by the sexual partner. Complications are rare. Prostatitis, littritis and cowperitis may be observed; balanitis and balano-posthitis occur mainly in uncircumcised subjects; cases of epididymitis and orchiepidymitis have been described [6-10].

3. Diagnosis

Positive diagnosis is based on fresh direct examination between slide and slide with staining (May-Grunwal Giemsa (MGG) stain or acidrine orange stain) [2]. Examination by staining is sufficient to make the diagnosis of *Trichomonas vaginalis* and lends itself easily to serial screening. Fresh direct examination has a sensitivity of 60-80% [11]. Culture on special media (Diamond, Roiron type) remains the reference technique, but requires a period of 3 to 7 days [11]. PCR (Polymerase Chain Reaction) techniques are performed on the first urine jet with excellent specificity [11, 12]. PCR is decisive in diagnosing asymptomatic forms. Some kits offer a combined PCR test for *N. gonorrhoeae, C. trachomatis and T. vaginalis* [12].

4. Treatment

Treatment of trichomoniasis is based on short courses of treatment and treatment of partners. It is based on nitroimidazoles: metronidazole 2g in one dose; miconazole; tinidazole [8, 13]. With the exception of metronidazole, these drugs are contraindicated in pregnancy. In the event of pregnancy, a local treatment may be proposed: metronidazole (ova). Resistance to these treatments has been reported in exceptional cases.

References

1. Freney J, Riegel P. Bacteriologie clinique 3[e] edition ESKA 2018
2. Janier M. Maladies sexuellement transmissibles, collection Abrege. Masson-Elsevier 2010
3. Hirt RP. Trichomonas vaginalis virulence factors: an integrative overview. Sex Transm Infect 2013;89:439-43.
4. Graves KJ, Ghosh AP, Kissinger PJ et al. *Trichomonas vaginalis:* a review of the literature. Int J STD AIDS 2019;30:496-504. .
5. Mabaso N, Abbai NS. A review on *Trichomonas vaginalis* infections in women from Africa. S Afr J Infect Dis 2021;36:254. doi: 10.4102/sajid.v36i1.254. eCollection 2021
6. Feleke DG, Yemanebrhane N. *Trichomonas vaginalis* infection in Ethiopia: A systematic review and meta-analysis. Int J STD AIDS 2022;33:232-241.
7. Rowley J, Vander-hoom S, Korenromp E et al. Chlamydia, gonorrheae, trichomiasis and syphilis. Global prevalence and incidence estimates. Bull Word health Organ 2019; 97: 548562
8. Centers for Diseases Control and Prevention. Sexually transmitted infections treatement. Guidelines 2021. MMR 2021; 70: 30-59
9. Edward T, Burke P, Smalley H, Hobbs G. *Trichomonas vaginalis*: Clinical relevance, pathogenicity and diagnosis. Crit Rev Microbiol 2016 :42:406-17.
10. Trei JS, Carres LC, Gould PL. Reproductive tract complications associated *Chlamydia trachomatis* infections in US Air Force males whithin 4 years testing. Sex Transm Dis 2008; 35: 827-33
11. Van Der Pol B. Clinical and Laboratory Testing for *Trichomonas vaginalis* infection. J Clin Microbiol. 2016 Jan;54(1):7-12. doi: 10.1128/JCM.02025-15
12. Hobbs MM, Sena AC Modern diagnosis of *Trichomonas vaginalis* infection. Sex Transm Infect. 2013; 89:434-8
13. Bouchema K, Bonies C, Loiseau PM. Strategies for prevention and treatement of *Trichomas vaginalis* infections. Clin Microbiol Rev 2017; 30 :811-25

Candida infection

1. Causal agent

It is a yeast of the genus Candida. The Candida genus comprises almost two hundred species [1]. The majority of Candida species are saprophytes of the skin, digestive tract and urogenital mucosa. *Candida albicans* subsp. *albicans* is the most frequently isolated species in digestive and genital diseases [1, 2]. Factors favouring the pathogenicity of *C. albicans* are host-related (immunodepression, neonates, pregnancy, perspiration) and exogenous (antibiotic therapy, long-term corticosteroid therapy, immunosuppressants, catheters) [3, 4].

In sexually active adults, candidiasis accounts for 15% of non-gonococcal urethral and vaginal infections [1, 2]. In women, the presence of *C. albicans* in vaginal secretions is not necessarily an STI.

2. Symptomatology

In women

- The most classic manifestation is acute vulvovaginitis, which combines three signs: vulvar pruritus, which is often violent and permanent; vaginal burning, causing dyspareunia or even preventing penetration; and abundant, whitish, thick, creamy leucorrhoea, with premenstrual recrudescence [5]. Clinical examination shows a very erythematous vulvar region, sometimes redematous. The lips are deformed and varnished. Lesions may extend beyond the vulva, the clitoris, the perineum, the perianal area, the gluteal fold and the metabolic area, causing dysuria. The vaginal mucosa is generally red with whitish granulations (vaginal thrush). Sometimes the vaginal and cervical mucosa are completely lined with creamy leucorrhoea.

- Vulvovaginitis sulxuguc' presents a simpler symptomatology: minimal vulvar lesions, scanty leucorrhoea, with moderate and intermittent pruritus [4, 5]. Chronic or recurrent vulvovaginitis evolves in flare-ups interspersed with periods of calm lasting a few weeks. In the long term, they interfere with a couple's sexual and emotional life. It is essential to look for a predisposing or triggering factor (immunodepression: long-term corticosteroid treatment, HIV, diabetes).

There are other forms of vulvovaginal candidiasis that are important to know about:

- Recurrent vulvovaginal candidiasis: this is defined as the occurrence of at least three episodes during the year. The risk factors for recurrence are not well documented (destruction of vaginal flora by unsuitable toilets? Immunocompromising conditions such as diabetes or HIV; individual susceptibility). In 10-20% of cases, *C. glabrata* or other non-albicans species are present [6, 7].
- Severe vulvovaginitis is characterised by extensive vulvar erythema, severe vaginal lip swelling, excoriations and fissures [8, 9]. Management requires longer local and general treatment (7 to 14 days).

In pregnant women, the frequency of genital candidiasis is increased, but there is no risk to the unborn child [6].

In men

The classic form of genital involvement is balanitis or balanoposthitis [1]. Balanitis begins as an erythematous macule on the glans penis. The lesions become generalised and coalesce into patches or blotches with a crumbling outline. Sensations of pruritus or burning are sometimes reported. The presence of candida in the semen of asymptomatic subjects raises the possibility of prostatic and/or vesicular localization.

3. Diagnosis

Positive diagnosis is based on direct microscopic examination of a drop of urethral or vaginal secretion, looking for mycelial filaments. A few drops of methylene blue or toluidine blue increase the sensitivity of the method. Cultures are essential to confirm the diagnosis, by isolating the species. In 80% of cases it is C. albicans subsp. albicans [10]. In cases of chronic or recurrent infection, or where there is a suspicion of treatment failure, an antifungiogram may be requested in order to suggest an improved treatment. The differential diagnosis is discussed clinically with the other causes of urethritis and vulvovaginitis: additional tests may help to resolve any clinical doubts.

Once the clinic and diagnosis have been made, a classification of candidiasis vulvovaginitis can be drawn up. This classification can help in the management and follow-up of patients.

Table 4: Classification of candidiasis vulvovaginitis (CVV) [9].

Uncomplicated VVC

- Sporadic, clinically moderate VVC due to C. *albicans*
- Female immunocompetence

Complicated VVC

- Recurrent CVV (at least three episodes in a year)
- Or VVC severe
- VVC due to Candida non albicans
- Or women with a history of diabetes or immunodepression (HIV, therapeutic immunosuppression)

4. Treatment

The treatment of urethrovaginal candidiasis is still largely dominated by local therapies and the thiazole class (ketoconazole, itraconazole, fluconazole) [3, 8, 9, 11].

In women. Ovules or gynaecological tablets of imidazole derivatives are used (for 3 to 6 days). A single oral fluconazole capsule (150 mg) gives excellent results with good therapeutic comfort. The search for and treatment of predisposing conditions and triggering factors potentiates the results of treatment and avoids the onset of chronicity or frequent recurrences.

In men. The treatment for balanitis combines cleansing with a mild soap and a local antimycotic treatment in cream or milk (econazole, isoconazole etc.). Associated urethritis is treated with fluconazole: a single 150 mg capsule. The search for an anatomical anomaly and its surgical cure will help prevent recurrence.

In both sexes. In cases of immunosuppression, frequent recurrence, chronicity or severity of the condition or VVC due to non-albicans Candida, systemic treatment should be offered as a first step, with simultaneous treatment of sexual partners and, above all, investigation and management of the contributing factors [9, 11].

References

1. Achkar JM, Fries BC. Candida infections of the genitourinary tract.Clin Microbiol Rev 2010;23:253-73.

2. Ohmit SE, Sobel JD, Schuman P et al. HIV epidemiology research study (HERS) group. Longitidunal study of mucosal Candida species colonization and candidiasis among human immunodeficieny virus seropositive and at-risk HIV-seronegative women ? J Infec Dis 2003; 188: 118-27

3. Mushi MF, R, Bongomin F. Prevalence, antifungal susceptibility and etiology of vulvovaginal candidiasis in sub-Saharan Africa: a systematic review with meta-analysis and meta-regression. Med Mycol 2022;60:myac037. doi: 10.1093/mmy/myac037.

4. Mtibaa L, Fakhfakh N, Kallel A et al. Vulvovaginal candidiasis: Etiology, symptomatology and risk factors. .J Mycol Med. 2017;27:153-158.

5. Duerr A, Heilig CM, Meikle SP et al. HER Study Group. Incident and persistent vulvovaginal candidiasis among HIV-infected women: risk factor and severity? Obstet Gynecol 2003 ;101 :548-56

1.1. enning DW, Knealz M, Sobel JD et al. Global burden of recurrent vulvoginal candidiasis: a systemic review. Lancet Infect Dis 2018 ;18 : e339-47

7. Kennedy MA, Sobel JD. Vulvovaginal candidiasis caused by on-albicancs Candida; new insignts. Curr Infec Dis Rep 2010; 12: 465-10

8. Sobet JD. Recurrent vulvovaginal candidiasis. Am J Obstet Gynecol 2016;214:15-21.

9. Sobel JD, Faro S, Force RW et al. Vulvoginal candidiasis: epidemiologic diagnostic and

therapeutic considerations. Am J Obstet Gynecol 1998 ;178 :203-11
10. Dermendzhiev T, Pehlivanov B, Petrova A et al. Quantitative system for diagnosis of vulvovaginal candidiasis. J Mycol Med. 2022;32:101302. doi: 10.1016/j.mycmed.2022.101302. Epub 2022
11. Centers for Diseases Control and Prevention. Sexually transmitted infections treatement. Guidelines 2021. MMR 2021; 70: 30-59

Bacterial vaginosis

Bacterial vaginosis is defined as "a condition in which the lactobacilli of the vagina are replaced by characteristic groups of bacteria and which results in a change in the properties of vaginal fluids" [1]. This is vaginal dysbiosis.

1. Causal agent

Vaginosis is an imbalance in the microbial flora of the vagina, characterised by the disappearance of lactobacilli and gram-positive bacteria and the multiplication of anaerobic germs such as Gardnerella vaginalis, Prevotellea spp and Mobiluncus spp [1, 2]. Lactobacilli are beneficial to the vaginal flora because they ensure an adequate level of acidity in the vagina, preventing pathogenic germs from developing. *Gardnerella vaginalis* is a common host in the vaginal flora, living in equilibrium with the other germs. This bacterium can sometimes cause infections of the female genital tract. The bacteria present in the vagina protect against infections in everyday life, but when there is a significant proliferation of a particular bacterium, we are in the presence of a vaginal infection [3]. The infection is generally endogenous. It involves the excessive proliferation of germs which, in small quantities, are part of the normal vaginal flora. However, there are arguments to support the transmissibility of *Gardnerella vaginalis* (the causative germ) [1, 2]: *i)* the presence of the germ in the partner's urethra and semen; *ii)* the high frequency of infection in patients attending STI clinics, in contrast to the rarity of infection in sexually inactive women [7, 8].

2. Symptomatology

In women. Vaginosis is characterised by a greyish, homogeneous, fluid leucorrhoea adherent to the vaginal walls, generally non-purulent, with an unpleasant odour ("rotten fish" smell); this odour is accentuated if a drop of 10% KOH solution is added to the discharge between slide and coverslip [1, 2]. Accompanying signs (burning, pruritus, dysuria) are more discreet than in trichomoniasis and vaginal candidiasis. Fetomaternal complications have been described rarely, and in immunocompromised patients [5, 6].

In men. In most cases, the infection is asymptomatic, although erythema and pruritus around the meat, urethritis or cystitis may occur in exceptional cases [4].

3. Diagnosis

Three of the following four criteria are essential to confirm the diagnosis of bacterial vaginosis [9] :

- increased quantity of homogeneous vaginal discharge ;
- characteristic "rotten fish" smell (potash test) ;
- Vaginal PH greater than 4.5
- fresh microscopic examination revealed the presence of rods adhering to epithelial cells, known as "clue-cells".

The diagnosis of vaginosis is not a diagnosis of exclusion, but is based on certain objective criteria. These criteria make it possible to rule out saprophytic or pathogenic germs that may cause leucorrhoea.

4. **Treatment**

Although the germ is sensitive to a number of antibiotics, the standard treatment remains metronidazole or its imidazole derivatives [10, 11]. The standard dose is 500 mg per day orally for seven days, or 2 g in 2 doses or as a single dose. In the event of contraindication (pregnant women in their first trimester). Treatment of the partner should only be considered in the event of recurrence [11].

References

1. Nelson DB, Hanlon S, Hassan S et al. Paternal labor and bacterial vaginosis-associated bacteria among urban women? J Perinat Med 2009; 37: 130-4

2. Muzny CA, Laniewski P, Schwebke JR, et al. Host-vaginal microbiota interactions in the pathogenesis of bacterial vaginosis. Curr Opin Infect Dis 2020;33:59-65.

3. Jung H, Ehlers MM, Peters RPH et al. Growth Forms of *Gardnerella* spp. and *Lactobacillus* spp. on Vaginal Cells. Front Cell Infect Microbiol. 2020 ;10:71. doi: 10.3389/fcimb.2020.00071.

4. Jung HS, Ehlers MM, Lombaard H et al. Etiology of bacterial vaginosis and polymicrobial biofilm formation. Crit Rev Microbiol. 2017;43:651-667.

5. Laxmi U, Agrawal S, Raghunandan C et al. Association of bacterial vaginosis with fetomaternal outcome in women wtih spontaneous preterm labor: prospective cohort study? J Matern Fetal Neonatal Med 2012; 25: 64-7

6. Gosmann C, Anathar MN, Handley SA et al. Lacobacillus-deficient cervicovaginal bacterial communities are associated with increased HIV acquisition in young South African women. Immunity 2017; 46 : 29-37

7. Coudray MS, Madhivanan P. Bacterial vaginosis-A brief synopsis of the literature. Eur J Obstet Gynecol Reprod Biol 2020;245:143-148.

8. ReidG. Is bacterial vaginosis a disease? Appl Microbiol Biotechnol 2018;102:553-558.

9. Africa CJW. Efficacy of methods used for the diagnosis of bacterial vaginosis. Expert Opin Med Diagn 2013;7:189-200.

10. Vodstrcil LA, Muzny CA, Plummer EL et al. Bacterial vaginosis: drivers of recurrence and challenges and opportunities in partner treatment. BMC Med 2021; 19:194. doi: 10.1186/s12916-021-02077-3.

11. Centers for Diseases Control and Prevention. Sexually transmitted infections treatement. Guidelines 2021. MMR 2021; 70: 30-59.

Genital infections caused by pyogenic germs

Several aerobic or anaerobic germs are found in genital discharges, but their sexually transmissible nature is uncertain. Some bacteria that are usually non-pathogenic may exceptionally cause urethritis [1, 2]: *Haemophilus influenzae, Haemophilus parainfluenzae, Staphylococcus saprohyticus, Streptococcus milleri, Bacteroides ureolyticus.* Acute meningococcal urethritis may be observed after oral sex in homosexuals [3], and *Escherichia coli* and streptococcal urethritis after anal sex. In these cases, the infection was discovered by chance on the results of cultures taken during a thorough work-up.

In men, certain bacteria are responsible for sulxugucous urethritis, the complications of which can be prostatitis or epididymal extension. In women, the infection is generally vulvar and is sometimes complicated by involvement of the Skene or Bartholin glands. In both sexes, particularly in men who have sex with men, pharyngeal and/or anorectal signs may be observed [3]. Management can be difficult, as it is necessary to distinguish between a pathogenic etiology and the discovery of germs that are *a priori* saprophytic or commensal to the genital tract. The interpretation of bacteriological results is sometimes difficult, and we must not hesitate to compare these results with the clinical context.

References

1. Holmred KK, Handsfield HH, Wang SP al. Etiology of nongonococcal urethritis. N Engl J Med 1975; 292: 1199-205.

2. Maini M, French P, Prince M, Bingham JS. Urethritis due to *Neisseria meningitidis* in a London genitourinary medicine clinic population. In J STD AIDS 1992; 2: 54-55

3. Barbee LA, Khosppour CM, Dombrowski JC et *al.* An estimate of proportion of symptomatic

gonococcal chlamydial and non-gonococcal on-chlamydial urethritis attributable to oral sex among men who have sex with sex men: a case control study. Sex Transm Infect 2016; 92: 155-60

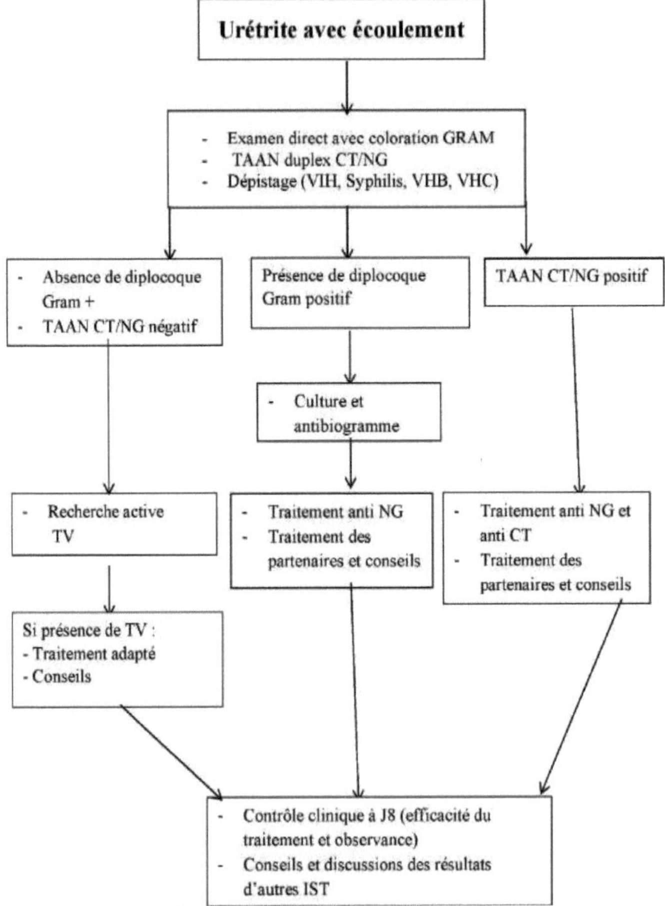

Figure 4: Treatment of a patient suffering from urethritis with discharge

Notes : NAAT: Nucleic Acid Amplification Test; NG: *Neisseria gonorrhoeae*; CT: *Chlamydia trachomatis;* TV: *Trichomonas vaginalis;* ECBU: Cytobacteriological Urine Examination; HIV: Human Immunodeficiency Virus; HBV: Hepatitis B virus; HCV: Hepatitis C virus; D8 (8th day)

PART III

III. Genital ulcers

Syphilis

1. Causal agent

Syphilis is a systemic infection caused by *Treponema pallidum* subsp *pallidum*, whose reservoir is exclusively human. *Treponema pallidum* subsp *pallidum* is a helicoidal bacillus identified in 1905 by Schauddin and Hoffman [1]. Treponemes belong to the order Spirochoerales. There are several species that are mucosal saprophytes. Only three species are pathogenic for humans. *Trepronema pallidum, Treponema pertenue* (agent of yaws), *Treponema carateun* (agent of pinta) [1-3].

Over the last two decades, there has been a resurgence of syphilis worldwide, particularly in Europe and the United States [4]. This resurgence is particularly marked among men who have sex with men (MSM) and people living with HIV [4-8].

2. Symptomatology

There is a consensus on the classification of syphilis. In addition to the old classification based on natural history into primary, secondary and tertiary stages, all learned societies and public health management organisations have adopted a more operational classification to ensure better management of syphilis [9, 10]. These are :

- early syphilis *(less than a year old),* which includes primary syphilis, secondary syphilis and early latent syphilis. This type of syphilis is characterised by a contagious phase with mainly mucocutaneous lesions. Neurological involvement is rare, and the prognosis is not life-threatening;
- late syphilis (*more than a year old), which* includes late latent syphilis and tertiary syphilis. This phase is not very contagious, but central nervous system involvement is common and can be life-threatening.

It should be noted that the WHO, while adopting this classification, has adopted slightly different timeframes: early syphilis (< 2 years); late syphilis (> 2 years).

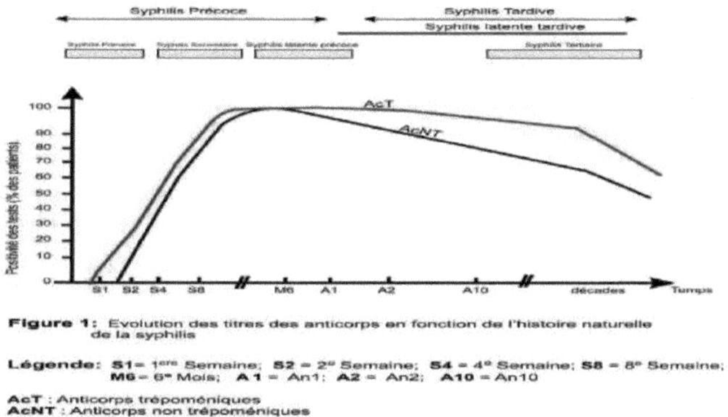

Figure 5: Natural history and classification of syphilis [10].

Early syphilis

Primary syphilis

After an incubation period ranging from 9 to 90 days (average 21 days), the first clinical manifestation of syphilis is marked by a chancre at the site of inoculation, accompanied by regional satellite adenopathy. The typical chancre is usually single, painless, pink in colour, with a regular, clean outline [10]. It gives the palp an impression of hard or cardboard-like consistency (hence the name hard chancre, as opposed to soft chancre).

- In men, the chancre sits on the balanopreputial groove, the sheath and the sub preputial frenulum - In women, the chancre (which is less and less common) sits on the large lips, small lips and the cervix or its papulo-erosive appearance can lead to it being confused with exo-cervicitis or endo-cervicitis.
- In both sexes, an extra-genital syphilitic chancre may be observed, particularly on the lips, fingers, oropharynx and anorectal region [11-13].

Atypical chancres may be observed [10]: syphilitic chancre may be multiple, sometimes painful (superinfectious chancre), sometimes ulcerous with a dirty background, and very inflammatory. It should be noted that syphilitic chancre and herpetic lesions may occur simultaneously (mixed chancre). If left untreated, the chancre will regress spontaneously after 3 weeks. Syphilitic chancre may mimic other ulcerative genital conditions [14]. Syphilitic chancre is accompanied by unilateral satellite adenopathy which is firm, painless and without periadenitis.

Secondary syphilis.

If left untreated, secondary syphilis develops between the sixth week and the third month. This is due to the systemic hematogenic spread of T. *pallidum.* Secondary syphilis often reveals the disease in women and MSM, in whom the chancre is rarely observed [9, 10]. Secondary syphilis is dominated by cutaneous and mucosal manifestations. Classically, a distinction is made between two blooming stages, according to the chronology of their appearance.

The first flowering is marked by the appearance of roseola. It appears in the form of non-itchy, non-infiltrated, purplish-coloured macules, mainly on the trunk. This rash must be distinguished from medical, food-related or infectious rashes. During the first bloom, mucosal lesions may be observed, consisting of macules with clear, rounded borders and a smooth, red colour. Mucosal lesions occur in the oral cavity (on the cheeks and gums, with involvement of the tongue giving the appearance of mown patches), on the labial commissures, on the vulva, and in the anal region, where they may be fissured or hypertrophic, simulating condylomas [15]. In addition to mucocutaneous involvement, alopecia may be observed in the clearing (between the third and sixth months), preferentially in the temporo-occipital region, especially retroauricular. In the case of recent alopecia in a young patient, a syphilitic serology should be performed [17].

The second flowering. It may be continuous with roseola or occur after a period of clinical latency between the fourth and twelfth months. It is characterised by the appearance of syphilis: rounded papules, rarely pruritic, protruding, infiltrated and pigmented [1, 10, 11, 18-20]. There are several types of syphilis.

- Lenticular papular or papulo-squamous syphilis occurs particularly in the flexion creases, palms and soles, labial commissures (syphilitic perch) and nasolabial folds.
- Papulo-erosive syphilis is common in the ano-genital region and in the folds.
- Papular syphilis appears on the trunk, face, labial commissures, scalp, face and chin.

In addition to skin manifestations, signs of hematopoietic organ and visceral involvement may be observed at this stage [1]. A painless generalized polyadenopathy without periadenitis, consisting of small firm lymph nodes, may be noted, with suggestive localizations (neck, elbow, epitrochlea). There may be visceral involvement, such as splenomegaly or hepatitis, which may be manifested by icterus or massive proteinuria, rarely meningitis, or osteitis with periostitis of the long bones, kneecaps and skull [21, 22]. Diagnosis of the second bloom is difficult because the lesions may mimic several dermatoses. Syphilis may mimic flat warts, lichen, seborrheic warts, psoriasis, leprosy or Gibert's pink pityriasis [14, 23].

Early latent syphilis

It is the chance discovery of a positive syphilitic serology in an asymptomatic subject that prompts the diagnosis [1]. Nowadays, this is the most common circumstance in which syphilis is discovered in practice. It may be due to antibiotic therapy prescribed for a trivial infection, which is insufficient for effective treatment of syphilis, or to unrecognised primary accidents (anorectal, cervical or oral chancre). Latent syphilis is said to be early if it is less than a year old [10]. In practice, serology can be difficult to interpret.

Late syphilis

Tertiary syphilis

After the secondary phase, untreated syphilis enters an asymptomatic period that can last for years or even decades (late latent syphilis) before the onset of tertiary syphilis: 5-10% of infected patients reach this phase [1]. It usually appears five to ten years after the primary infection (between 2 and 30 years). However, since the advent of penicillin and widespread access to antibiotics, these manifestations have become exceptional. The clinical signs of tertiary syphilis are dominated by cutaneous, skeletal, cardiovascular and neurological disorders.

Cutaneous and osseous manifestations: these are syphilitic gums [1, 9, 10]. These are papulo-nodular dermo-hypodermal lesions of variable size, sometimes annular in shape. Involvement of the mucous membranes may lead to erosions, ulceration or fistulisation, resulting in the destruction of certain mucous membranes. The erosion of a cutaneous or subcutaneous gum may lead to an ulcer with vertical edges, which may result in destruction of the mucosa (destruction of the cartilage of the nasal septum). Bone gums cause focal areas of disjunction and can erode cortical surfaces, leading to fractures and sometimes joint destruction [23]. Cutaneous and bony gumming should prompt discussion of cutaneous tuberculosis, deep-seated mycosis, sarcoidosis or leishmaniasis.

Cardiovascular syphilis. This is one of the life-threatening clinical manifestations of tertiary syphilis, but has become rare nowadays [28]. Signs of angina pectoris (due to occlusion of the coronary ostia), aortic insufficiency (due to enlargement and incontinence of the aortic valve) and aortic aneurysm formation may be observed [24].

Neurosyphilis. Neurosyphilis, ocular syphilis and otitis are secondary to treponemal invasion of the central nervous system. Neurosyphilis is relatively rare and is more common in MSM and people living with HIV [25]. The symptoms of general paralysis are most precocious, resulting in diffuse meningoencephalitis. It is characterised by a psychiatric syndrome (irritability, mood disorders, dementia) and a neurological syndrome (tremors of the limbs, dysarthria with the presence of the Argyll-Robertson sign in 50% of cases). Tabes appears later, after several years. It involves disorders of deep sensibility, responsible for ataraxia and searing pain. The Argyll-Robertson sign is more common (70-80%) [1, 19, 25]. Trophic disorders, plantar perforation pain and osteoarthropathy may also be observed. The clinical picture of neurosyphilis is currently dominated by signs of chronic meningitis (persistent headache, asthenia, personality disorders) or meningo-encephalitis, which may be accompanied by comitial seizures and damage to the cranial nerves (particularly III, VI, VII and VIII). Ocular or auricular involvement may be isolated or form part of the neurosyphilis picture with the presence of other signs [10, 25]. Ocular syphilis may present as retinitis or uveitis with visual disturbances. Ear involvement is characterized by a decrease or partial or total loss of hearing.

Congenital syphilis

Transmission of *T. pallidum* from mother to child can occur throughout pregnancy (rarely at delivery or during breast-feeding), which is why it is so important to carry out syphilis tests at the antenatal clinic [1, 10]. If the test is positive in a pregnant woman, ultrasound monitoring is required throughout the pregnancy, at birth and even during breast-feeding, in addition to appropriate treatment. Classically, a distinction is made between early congenital syphilis and late congenital syphilis.

Congenital syphilis occurs from birth to two years of age. At the time of birth, two symptoms may attract attention: *i)* low birth weight and the "appearance of a little old man"; *ii)* the placenta is enlarged, weighing more than 1/6 of the child's weight. Clinical signs are dominated by intense coryza, red stomatitis, skin rash, icterus, osteochondritis of the long bones, periostitis, hepatosplenomegaly and renal damage [9].

Late-onset congenital syphilis is currently exceptional in most countries. It is seen after the age of two, more often between the ages of 5 and 10, and sometimes later. It is due to the absence of early manifestations that did not attract the attention of family and friends at birth, or to the existence of undetected latent forms. Clinical signs include chorioretinitis, interstitial keratitis, deafness, Hutchinson's teeth, hydarthrosis of the knee, mucocutaneous gums (including palatal perforation) and neurological signs.

Syphilis and HIV infection

The relationship between syphilis and HIV infection is close. More than 50% of precocious syphilis cases in Europe and the United States occur in people living with HIV, particularly in seropositive MSM [1, 9, 10]. Syphilis is a marker of high-risk sexuality in both homosexuals and heterosexuals, and a history of syphilis increases the likelihood of having been exposed to HIV. There is no evidence that syphilis alters the natural history of HIV infection; however, HIV infection does alter the natural history of syphilis. There is an increased frequency of chancres during the primary phase, with chronic chancres associated with the eruption of secondary syphilis [23]. The onset of serious complications (ocular and neurological damage) appears to be more frequent and, above all, more precocious in the immunocompromised than in the healthy subject [25].

3. Diagnosis

Positive diagnosis.

Direct examinations

Dark-field microscopy. It consists of detecting T. *pallidum* in lesions. Direct detection is only carried out in lesions of primary and secondary syphilis (chancre, lymph nodes, mucous plaques); it can also be carried out on bullous lesions of congenital syphilis [26].

Direct immunofluorescence on a slide reveals green-coloured treponemes that are not deformed but immobile. This technique has good sensitivity but requires suitable equipment and trained staff [27].

The molecular amplification technique (PCR). It is increasingly used, with sensitivity and specificity for primary and secondary syphilis ranging from 80 to 96% and 96 to 100% respectively [9, 26]. This sensitivity is low in latent and late syphilis [53].

Culture and histology. T. pallidum cannot be cultured in practice, but is cultured from rabbit orchites in the laboratory [26]. Histology of lesions (syphilis and gum) is variable, non-specific and shows a perivascular dermal infiltrate rich in plasma cells. Histology may also show a gigantocellular epithelioid granuloma in gum lesions [49]. ***Serological tests***

Serological tests are the most practical because of the fugacity of the chancre and the inconsistency of secondary lesions. Antibodies appear between 5[eme] and 12[eme] days after the onset of the chancre. The serological tests currently available are fairly effective. Current treponemal tests have very good sensitivity and specificity for the diagnosis of syphilis [26-29].

Non-specific serological reactions or non-treponemal tests (NTT).

They use cardiolipid antigens common to treponemes and spirochetes. This type of test is positive between 10 and 15 days after the appearance of the chancre. This is the classic *VDRL* (*Venereal Diseases Research Laboratories*) or VDRL anthrax reaction. A variant is the Rapid Plasma Reagin (RPR) or Toluidine Red Unheated Serum Test (TRUST). These serological tests are suitable for mass screening. Titers peak during the secondary phase and then decline slowly and progressively, sometimes becoming negative after several years. Many false positives have been observed during various antigenic stimuli: pregnancy, connective tissue diseases, drug addiction, bacterial and viral infections [23].

Specific serological reactions or treponemal tests (TT). They are positive between 5[e] and 15[e] days after the appearance of the chancre.

- TPHA (Treponema Pallidum Haemagglutination Assay). TPHA is a hemagglutination of sheep red blood cells coated with treponemal antigen. False positives are extremely rare. Titers rapidly peak during the secondary phase, but decline very slowly, even under treatment (so TPHA is not a good test for monitoring treated syphilis).
- FTA (Fluorescent Treponemal Antibody). The simple or absorbed FTA on *Treponema reiteri* is a highly sensitive, highly specific immunofluorescence test on treponemal, but requires a laboratory that carries out immunofluorescence tests. The FTA is the first treponemal test to become positive between days 5^e^ and 10^e^ of the chancre. Titers peak in the secondary phase and then decline progressively but much more slowly than VDRL titres. Anti-treponemal IgM can be detected using an anti-IgM test. This test is important in screening for meningeal syphilis and in congenital syphilis. A positive FTA-IgM is an indication of active infection, but does not prejudge the age of the infection.
- Nelson test (Treponema Pallidum Immobilization Test: TPI). This is the treponemal immobilisation test and requires the use of rabbits. The Nelson test is by far the most specific serological reaction for syphilis and other treponematoses. Because of its extreme specificity, the Nelson test is the arbiter of contentious diagnoses (discrepancies between non-treponemal and treponemal serological reactions, and between clinical and biological data). It is not commonly used (it is used as a test of last resort in certain cases).
- Immonoenzymatic tests: ELISA (Enzyme Linked Immuno-Sorbent Assay) or EIA (Enzyme Immuno-Assay) or Chemi-Luminescence Immuno-Assay (CLIA) and immunoblot. ELISA/EIA/CLIA tests use processed recombinant *T. pallidum* antigens and are mostly automated and fairly standardised. They have very good sensitivity and specificity, and are capable of detecting antibodies from 5^e^ days after the chancre [26].

Diagnostic approach

Screening for syphilis. It is recommended to combine qualitative treponemal tests (ELISA/EIA/CLIA) and non-treponemal tests (RPR or VDRL) [30].

Confirmation of the diagnosis. In the event of positive screening, it is important to perform a quantitative assay of non-treponemal tests and treponemal tests on the same serum before starting any treatment [30]. However, despite the performance and automation of the majority of serological tests, and given the natural history of syphilis, biologists and, above all, clinicians may encounter a number of eventualities.

- ***TNT (-) TT (-):*** in principle, syphilis can be ruled out. However, the patient may have recently been infected (visible chancre or not). To rule out syphilis, FTA-Abs should be performed with IgM testing, or a new serology should be performed 10 to 15 days later (especially in high-risk patients), as antibodies do not appear in syphilis patients for 5 days.
- ***TNT (+) TT (+)****:* This is very likely to be active syphilis or active or recently cured endemic treponematosis (check the patient's origin or look for a history of residence in an endemic area). The history and clinical examination, supported by additional quantitative tests, will help to define the stage and evolution of the infection detected. IgM is always positive in primary and secondary syphilis. Levels peak between the third and sixth months.
- ***TNT (-) TT (+):*** this is either precocious active syphilis (chancre within the first five days) or old syphilis that has been treated and cured. This second situation is often considered to be a serological scar. The indication for treatment will depend essentially on the clinical cardiovascular and neurological examination, which may or may not show the existence of late syphilis. In all cases of discordance, the examination should be repeated after two weeks, especially in certain at-risk individuals (MSM, PLHIV) and pregnant women.
- ***TNT (+) TT (-):*** this is probably a false-positive cardiolipid reaction, so syphilis must be ruled out. These false positive VDRL reactions are found in a number of pathological or physiological situations: pregnancy; vaccination; infectious diseases or autoimmune diseases.

Differential diagnosis

Syphilis is a great simulator at all stages of the disease (primary syphilis, secondary syphilis and tertiary syphilis) (Tab.5).

Table 5: Diagnostic differentials in syphilis

Events	Differential diagnosis
Primary syphilis chancre	Infections Herpes, chancre mou Venereal lymphogranulomatosis Donovanose Sign pox Non-infectious conditions Traumatic ulceration Mouth ulcers Behcet's disease Bullous toxidermia Squamous cell carcinoma Zoon's barnacle
Secondary syphilis rash	Trunk locations Viral maculopapular exanthems Sign pox Medicated maculopapular exanthema Psoriasis, Gibert's pink pityriasis Flat warts, seborrheic dermatitis Lichen Palmar location Erythema multiforme Hand-foot syndrome
Gums for tertiary syphilis	Leprosy, leishmaniasis Deep mycoses (histoplasmosis type) Sarcoidosis
False positive serology (non-treponemal serology)	Infections Hepatitis, tuberculosis, leprosy, toxoplasmosis, mononucleosis Other causes Connectivites, Myeloma Pregnancy, Behcet's disease

4. Treatment

The curative treatment of syphilis, whatever its clinical form, stage or terrain, is based on penicillin, whose consistent efficacy makes it the reference treatment [31, 32]. Only if it is contraindicated should other antibiotics be used.

Therapeutic means

Penicillin. Benzathine penicillin G: this is packaged in 2.4 million units or 1.2 million units and is used intramuscularly (IM). In addition to Benzathine penicillin, procaine penicillin is also available in 600,000 to 1.2 million units for IM use. Penicillin G is the only form that can be used intravenously, and comes in 1 to 5 million units. The side effects of penicillin are essentially allergies, severe forms of which are a contraindication to its use. In view of their efficacy, some authors suggest desensitisation to penicillin [32].

Other antibiotics. These are an alternative when penicillin is contraindicated. Several studies have demonstrated the efficacy of doxycycline and ceftriaxone in the treatment of syphilis [33, 34]. Doxycycline is offered at 200 mg per day. Its use is contraindicated during pregnancy and in children. However, doxycycline does not spread well in the meninges. Ceftriaxone: 1g intravenously. Its efficacy and good meningeal distribution make it a good alternative to penicillin in neurosyphilis. Macrolides and related drugs (erythromycin and azithromycin) are no longer recommended for the treatment of syphilis because of their low level of efficacy due to the appearance of genomic resistance [30, 31, 34].

Indications [31, 32].

Recent syphilis (less than 1 year old). Benzathine penicillin G (BPG) is administered intramuscularly in a single dose of 2.4 million units (or an injection of 1.2 MIU into each buttock). In the event of allergy to penicillin, doxycycline 200 mg per day *orally* for 14 days is suggested. In

the event of allergy to penicillin and contraindication to cyclins, there are two alternatives: either ceftriaxone 1g per day IV for 10 days, or penicillin desensitisation.
Late syphilis (excluding neurosyphilis). Benzathine penicillin G: 2.4 million units per week for 3 weeks or procaine penicillin 600,000 units IM per day for 21 days. In the event of an allergy to penicillin, a lumbar puncture is essential and the patient must be examined.
conditions treatment. If CSF is present, the recommended alternative is doxycycline (200 mg per day for 21 to 28 days). If biological meningitis is present, it should be treated as neurosyphilis.
Neurosyphilis, ocular and auricular syphilis. Penicillin G: 18 to 24 million units per day intravenously (i.e. 3 to 4 million units every 4 hours) for 10 to 14 days. Only intravenous penicillin G guarantees a treponemic concentration in the CSF. In the event of allergy to penicillin, there is no very effective alternative. Either penicillin desensitisation must be performed, or ceftriaxone 1-2 g per day IV for 10-14 days. Recovery is judged by the reduction or disappearance of pleocytosis at 6^e months and 2 years.
Syphilis in pregnant women. Treatment is based on penicillin at a dosage appropriate to the stage of syphilis. As cyclins are contraindicated during pregnancy, in the event of allergy to penicillin, desensitisation should be offered, followed by the appropriate penicillin regimen.
Congenital syphilis. Penicillin G: 150,000 Ul/kg IV (in six doses every six hours) for 10-14 days or procaine penicillin 50,000 unites/kg/d in one intramuscular injection for 10 to 14 days.
Syphilis acquired during HIV infection. Penicillin remains the standard treatment as in non-HIV-infected patients, and the regimen will be adapted according to the clinical stages of the syphilis.
Jarish-Herxheimer reaction. It generally occurs within 24 hours of treatment and is more frequent during treatment with penicillin than with doxycycline [35]. It is common during treatment of early syphilis, probably because of the high bacterial load [36]. Clinical symptoms include fever, headache, myalgias and sometimes dyspnoea and hypotension. This reaction is often transient and does not constitute an allergy to penicillin. It is benign except in pregnant women, in whom it may trigger precocious labour and fatal suffering during pregnancy (it can be prevented by prescribing paracetamol or even prednisone, 0.5 mg/kg the day before and for the first 3 days) [31].

References

1. Hook EW. Syphilis. Lancet 2017;389:1550-1557.
2. Ghanem KG, Ram S, Rice PA. The Modern Epidemic of Syphilis. N Engl J Med 2020; 382:845-854
3. Fraser CM, Norris JS, Weinstock GM et al. Complete genome sequence of *Treponema pallidum,* the syphilis spirochete. Science 1998; 281:375-88
4. Spiteri G, Unemo M, Mardh O, Amato-Gauci AJ. The resurgence of syphilis in high-income countries in the 2000s: a focus on Europe. Epidemiol Infect 2019;147:e143
5. Newman L, Rowley J, Vander Hoorn S et al. Global estimates of the prevalence and incidence of four curable sexually transmitted infections in 2012 based on systematic review and global reporting. PLoS One 2015;10: e0143304
6. Hope-Rapp E, Anyfantakis V, Fouere S et al. Etiology of genital ulcer disease. A prospective study of 248 cases in Paris. Sex Transm Dis 2010;37:153-8.
7. European Centre for Disease Prevention and Control. Syphilis-annual epidemiological report for 2018. https://www.edc.europa.en/en/publications-data/syphilis-annual-epidemiological- report-2018
8. Abara WE, Hess KL, Neblett-Fanfair R et al. Syphilis Trends among Men Who Have Sex with Men in the United States and Western Europe: A Systematic Review of Trend Studies Published between 2004 and 2015. PLoS One 2016 22; 11: e0159309.
9. Eenschlager S. Cutaneous manifestations of syphilis: recognition and management. Am J Clin Dermatol. 2006;7:291-304
10. Forrestel AK, Kovarik CL, Katz KA. Sexually acquired syphilis: Historical aspects, microbiology, epidemiology, and clinical manifestations. J Am Acad Dermatol 2020, 82:1-14.

11. Ma DL, Vano-Galvan S. Images in clinical medicine. Annular secondary syphilis. N Engl J Med 2014;371: 2017
12. Leao JC, Gueiros LA, Porter SR. Oral manifestations of syphilis. Clinics 2006; 61:161-6
13. Ramfrez-Amador V, Anaya-Saavedra G, Crabtree-Ramfrez B et al. Clinical spectrum of oral secondary syphilis in HIV-infected patients. J Sex Transm Dis 2013; 2013:892427
14. Balagula Y, Mattei PL, Wisco OJ et al. The great imitator revisited: the spectrum of atypical cutaneous manifestations of secondary syphilis.CInt J Dermatol. 2014;53:1434-41
15. Shinkuma S, Abe R, Nishimura M et al. Secondary syphilis mimicking warts in an HIVpositive patient. Sex Transm Infect 2009; 85:484.
16. Ho EL, Lukehart SA. Syphilis: using modern approaches to understand an old disease. J Clin Invest 2011;121:4584-92
17. Lee JW, Jang WS, Yoo KH et al. Diffuse pattern essential syphilitic alopecia: an unusual form of secondary syphilis. Int J Dermatol 2012; 51:1006-7
18. Jaiswal AK, Bhardwaj M, Singh G et al. Palmoplantar syphilis: an isolated and identical manifestation of conjugal infection in marital partners.Int J Dermatol1994;33:449-50
19. Pandhi D, Reddy BS, Khurana N et al. Nodular syphilis mimicking histoid leprosy. J Eur Acad Dermatol Venereol 2005;19:256-7
20. Pourmanas CC, Masouye I, Pileta P et al. Extensive annular verrucous late secondary syphilis. Br J Dermatol 2005; 152:1343-1345
21. Park KH, Lee MS, Hong IK, et al. Bone involvement in secondary syphilis: a case report and systematic review of the literature. Sex Transm Dis 2014;41:532-7.
22. Kahn MF, Baillet R, Amouroux J et al. Subacute inflammatory rheumatism in secondary syphilis. Rev Rhumatol 1970;37:431-6
23. Pitche P. Sexually transmitted ulcerations. EMC-Dermatologie 2022; 24: 1-5 [article 98-450-A-10].
24. Landry T, Smyczek P, Cooper R Et al. Retrospective review of tertiary and neurosyphilis cases in Alberta, 1973-2017. BMJ Open 2019; 9:e025995.
25. Ropper AH. Neurosyphilis. N Engl J Med 2019;381:1358-1363.
26. Park IU, Tran A, Pereira L et al. Sensitivity and Specificity of treponemal-specific tests for the diagnosis of syphilis. Clin Infect Dis 2020;71(Suppl 1):S13-S20
27. Young H, Pryde J, Duncan L et al. The Architect syphilis assay for antibodies to Treponema pallidum: an automated screening assay with high sensitivity in primary syphilis. Sex Transm Infect 2009; 85:19-23
28. Marks M, Yin YP, Chen XS et al. Metaanalysis of the performance of a combined treponemal and nontreponemal rapid diagnostic test for syphilis and Yaws. Clin Infect Dis 2016; 63:627-633
29. Cole MJ, Perry KR, Parry JV. Comparative evaluation of15 serological assays for the detection of syphilis infection. Eur J Clin Microbiol Infect Dis 2007; 26:705-13
30. Tuddenham S, Katz SS, Ghanem KG. Syphilis laboratory guidelines: Performance characteristics of nontreponemal antibody tests. Clin Infect Dis 2020;71(Suppl 1):S21-S42
31. Janier M, Uemo U, Dupin N et al. 2020 European guidlines of management of syphilis. J Eur Acad Dermatol Venereol 2021; 35: 574-588
32. Centers for Diseases Control and Prevention. Sexually transmitted infections treatement. Guidelines 2021. MMR 2021; 70: 30-59
33. Chen JR, Tarver SA, Alvarez KS, et al. A Proactive approach to penicillin allergy testing in hospitalized patients. J Allergy Clin Immunol Pract 2017;5:686-693
34.. Liu HY, Han Y, Chen XS, et al. Comparison of efficacy of treatments for early syphilis: A systematic review and network meta-analysis of randomized controlled trials and observational studies. PLoS One 2017;12:e0180001
35. Tsai MS, Yang CJ, Lee NY et al. Jarisch-Herxheimer reaction among HIV-positive patients with early syphilis: azithromycin versus benzathine penicillin G therapy. J Int AIDS

Soc2014;17:18993
36. Arando M, Fernandez-Naval C, Mota-Foix M et al. The Jarisch-Herxheimer reaction in syphilis: could molecular typing help to understand it better? J Eur Acad Dermatol Venereol 2018; 32:1791-1795

Genital herpes

1. Causal agent

The causative agent of herpes is *Herpes simplex virus (HSV)*. HSV belongs to the Herpesviridae family, which are DNA viruses with at least fifty species [1]. *Herpes simplex* has two subtypes, HSV 1 and HSV 2, and humans are the only reservoir of HSV [1, 2].

Genital herpes is most often caused by infection with HSV2, but currently more than 35% of genital herpes are caused by HSV1, due to orogenital practices [3]. This is a common disease, as one adult in 5 is a carrier of this virus. However, epidemiological studies show that there is a large discrepancy between the prevalence of antibodies against herpes types 1 and 2 and clinically observed infection [4]. HSV type 2 can be transmitted through a number of different routes during heterosexual or homosexual activity. The factors associated with HSV 2 infection are high-risk sexual behaviour (in particular, a high number of sexual partners and failure to use condoms) and, for HSV 1, orogenital practices [5, 6].

2. Symptomatology

There are two types of clinical manifestation: primary and recurrent [7, 8]. However, it should be emphasised that, in practice, there is significant asymptomatic secretion in carriers of HSV infection, and it is this asymptomatic secretion that is a major factor in the transmission and spread of the virus [9].

Primary herpes infection

The incubation period for a primary infection is generally 7 to 21 days after the infecting intercourse. The existence of oral HSV $herpes_1$ does not protect against genital HSV $infection_2$ [1]. The first episode of genital herpes is accompanied by fever, headache, malaise and myalgia shortly after the onset of infection. These signs persist for three or four days, then subside and disappear. Genital signs often begin with paresthesia, pruritus or burning sensations on the genital teguments [1, 8, 10]. Lesions predominate in the vulvar and perineal region in women, with pain during intercourse or clinical examination, and the sheath and glans in men. The initial lesions are the classic cluster of vesicles on an erythematous base. These lesions may extend to the thighs and buttocks. The vesicles develop either directly into erosions or confluent ulcerations, or into bullae through coalescence and then ulceration. These ulcerations heal between one and two weeks without scarring. In men, the vesicular lesions are located on the sheath and are less painful [1]. In both sexes, pharyngeal and anal localisations can be observed [11, 12]. Localisations manifest as anorectal pain, rectitis, anal discharge or reflex constipation [10].

Local signs are accompanied by satellite inguinal adenopathy. In the case of mucosal lesions (cervical or urethral), vaginal and urethral discharge may be observed. Extra-genital localisations may be observed through auto-inoculation (buttocks, scrotum, thighs, fingers, eyes).

Recurrent genital herpes

Two-thirds of patients with a primary herpes infection will develop a recurrence within a year [2]. There are probably a large number of triggering factors: menstruation; intercurrent infection; fever; local skin trauma (frequent cuts); asthenia; heat; stress [2, 7]. In approximately 50% of cases, prodromal signs precede the appearance of mucocutaneous lesions by 24 to 48 hours. These include paresthesia, cutaneous hyperesthesia, pruritus, and burning, usually on or near the lesion site. An erythematous macule or plaque then rapidly appears, topped by a cluster of vesicles. This vesicular stage is rarely seen, and it is at the erosive stage that most patients seek help. The average duration is 6 to 7 days. The topography is exclusively genital and the symptoms are less noisy than those of primary infection. The rate of recurrence is higher for HSV_2 (95% of cases) than for HSV_1 (50-60% of cases) [3]. Herpes recurrence can have a significant psychosocial impact on patients. Recurrent symptoms of genital herpes can be painful and the infection can lead to social stigmatisation and psychological distress. These factors can have a major impact on quality of life and sexual relationships.

Herpes and HIV infection

In the course of HIV infection, severe forms are observed with extensive, delabridging lesions, evolving in a single course with no tendency for spontaneous healing, and requiring prolonged treatment with aciclovir. Chronic, extensive, genital herpes has a very high positive predictive value (95%) for HIV infection and is classified as AIDS [5].

Neonatal herpes

Newborns become infected at the time of birth, either when the membranes rupture or when they pass through the infected maternal birth canal. The risk of contamination in the event of maternal infection at term varies from 5 to 50% depending on the case [2, 8]. The virus can be transmitted *in utero,* perpartum and postpartum. It should be emphasised that in the majority of cases, transmission occurs at the time of delivery [2, 8, 10], and the risk of contamination of the child is all the greater in that it is the mother's first infection. Symptoms are dominated by neurological involvement (meningo-encephalitis), which appears during the second week of the newborn's life [11, 12]. The disseminated form (approximately 10%), with polyvisceral involvement (liver, lung, kidney) often associated with neurological involvement, is fatal in more than 80% of cases [12]. Hence the importance of systematically monitoring and treating episodes of herpes in pregnant women. Some studies recommend vaginal delivery in the event of a recent episode of genital herpes in the mother, particularly at the time of labour [11].

3. Diagnosis

Diagnosis is based on isolation of HSV1 or HSV2 in cell culture and PCR [13, 14]. Cell culture is the reference technique, enabling identification of the viral type. It should be emphasised that the sensitivity and specificity of culture depend in part on the quality of the clinical sample and the type of vesicular or crusted lesions [7]. PCR (Polymerase Chain Reaction) provides a rapid positive diagnosis with good sensitivity, and can also be used to diagnose the species through HSV-1/HSV-2 genotyping. PCR is a good tool in the case of asymptomatic secretions [12, 15]. Serology can be used to identify HSV antibody carriers, but is not suitable for the positive diagnosis of clinical lesions.

Genital herpes is differentially diagnosed with other causes of genital ulceration, particularly sexually transmitted (chancroid, syphilis, lymphogranulomatosis venereum, donovanosis) [16, 17].

4. Treatment

Treatment is with aciclovir or valaciclovir, antiviral drugs that have been shown to be effective, but which are virostatic and do not eradicate the infection [7, 18, 19].

Primary infection: oral aciclovir 1g/d (200 mg x 5) for 7 to 10 days or valaciclovir 1g/d (500 mg x 2/d) for 10 days.

Recurrent herpes: administration of aciclovir or valaciclovir tablets (1g per day for 5 days) accelerates healing and reduces the duration of viral excretion, especially if this treatment is given early. For the prevention of recurrences (patients with at least 6 recurrences per year), treatment with oral valaciclovir 500 mg once daily is recommended for a minimum of 12 months. The effectiveness of this prophylaxis should be assessed after one year. Aciclovir is thought to reduce the recurrence of HSV2 genital herpes at the time of treatment. In fact, long-term treatment reduces the frequency of recurrences during treatment, but has no effect on recurrences after the drug has been stopped [7].

Herpes in pregnant women: some authors recommend the prophylactic use of aciclovir (400 mg x 2/d) from 36^{e} weeks gestation in women who have had a first episode of genital herpes during pregnancy (but the effectiveness is debatable). Prophylactic cesarean section is recommended in the event of an outbreak of herpes at the time of labour [7]. Given the risk of contamination, cesarean section is indicated in the event of an outbreak of genital herpes in a woman at the time of labour.

Neonatal herpes: in cases of neonatal herpes, aciclovir and vidarabine are indicated. However, despite treatment, the prognosis for neonatal herpes is guarded [20].

References

1. Omarova S, Cannon A, Weiss W et al. Genital Herpes Simplex Virus-An Updated Review. Adv Pediatr 2022;69:149-162.
2. Gupta R, Warren T, Wald A. Genital herpes. Lancet 2007;370:2127-37
3. Ryder N, Jin F, McNulty AM et al. Increasing role of herpes simplex virus type 1 in first-episode anogenital herpes in heterosexual women and younger men who have sex with men, 1992-2006. Sex Transm Infect 2009;85:416-9.
4. Malkin JE, Morand P, Malvy D, Ly TD, Chanzy B, de Labareyre C, El Hasnaoui A, Hercberg S. Seroprevalence of HSV1 and HSV2 infection in the general French population. Sex Transm Infect 2002;78 :201-3
5. Kularatne RS, Muller EE, Maseko DV et al.Trends in the relative prevalence of genital ulcer disease pathogens and association with HIV infection in Johannesburg, South Africa, 20072015. PLoS One. 2018: 4;13(4):e0194125.doi: 10.1371/journal.pone.0194125.
6. Zetola NM, Bernstein KT, Wong E et al. Exploring the relationship between sexualy transmitted diseases and HIV acquisition by using different study designs. J Acquir Immune Defic Syndr 2009; 50: 546-51
7. Milpied B, Janier M, Timsit J et al. Genital herpes Ann Dermatol Venereol 2016 ;143:729-733
8. Grann JW Jr, Whitley RJ. Genital herpes. Clinical pratice. N Engl J Med 2016; 375; 66670
9. Wald A, Zeh J, Selke S et al. Virologic characteristic of subclinical and symptomatic genital herpes infections. N Engl J Med 1995;333:770-5.
10. Cole S. Herpes Simplex Virus: Epidemiology, Diagnosis, and Treatment. Nurs Clin North Am 2020;55:337-345.
11. Van Wagoner N, Qushair F, Johnston C. Genital Herpes Infection: Progress and problems. Infect Dis Clin North Am 2023;37:351-367.
12. Garland SM, Steben M. Genital herpes. Best Pract Res Clin Obstet Gynaecol. 2014;28:1098-110.
13. Wald A, Zeh J, Selke S et al. Virologic characteristic of subclinical and symptomatic genital herpes infections. N Engl J Med 1995; 333:770-5.
14. Wald A. Huang ML, Carrell D et al. Polymerase chain reaction for detection of herpes simplex virus (HSV) DNA on mucosal surfaces: comparison HSV isolation in cel culture. J Infect Dis 2003;18:1345-51
15. Jin J. Screening for Genital Herpes. JAMA 2023;329:520. doi: 10.1001/jama.2023.0454.
16. Pitche P. Sexually transmitted ulcerations. EMC-Dermatologie 2022; 24 : 1-5 [article 98-450-A-10].
17. Johnston C. Diagnosis and Management of genital herpes: Key questions and review of the evidence for the 2021 Centers for Disease Control and Prevention Sexually Transmitted Infections Treatment Guidelines. Clin Infect Dis 2022;74(Suppl_2):S134-S143.
18. Le Cleach L, Trinquart L, Do G et al. Oral antiviral therapy for prevention of genital herpes outbreaks in immunocompetent and non-pregnant patients. Cochrane Database Syst Rev. 2014;(8):CD009036. doi: 10.1002/14651858.CD009036.
19. Patel R, Kennedy OJ, Clarke E et al. 2017 European guidelines for the management of genital herpes. Int J STD AIDS. 2017;28:1366-1379
20. Hammad WAB, Konje JC. Herpes simplex virus infection in pregnancy - An update. Eur J Obstet Gynecol Reprod Biol 2021; 259:38-45.

Soft canker

1. Pathogen

The causative agent is a small Gram-negative bacillus called *Haemophilus ducreyi,* described by Ducrey in 1889 [1]. H. *ducreyi* is a homogenous species belonging to the genus Haemophilus. It is a bacterium adapted to humans and has not been described in the external environment or in animals. Chancre mou is a highly contagious, self-inoculating, cosmopolitan disease, most commonly found in tropical areas. It is much more common in men than in women: 20 men for every woman, but women are often asymptomatic carriers [2]. It is a germ that is currently being observed less and less, and studies suggest that chancre mou is in the process of being eliminated worldwide [3, 4].

2. Symptomatology

In humans. Classically, the characteristics of soft chancre are point by point opposed to those of syphilitic chancre (hard chancre). The incubation period is short: 2 to 5 days. The chancre begins as an inflammatory papule that rapidly leads to ulceration. This is a round or oval ulceration of variable diameter, very painful, with a sunken, dirty, purulent base and no indurated base [5-7]. The lesion is usually located on the shaft of the penis, but the soft chancre is usually multiple (self-inoculation of the germ) and other ulcerations can be seen on the pubis, scrotum and inner thighs. Inflammatory adenopathy occurs in over 50% of cases. It is painful and may suppurate spontaneously, progressing to fistulisation and even chancrellisation with loss of substance [8, 9].

In women. Chancre is rare. It occurs on the large lips and in the region of the fork and, in this case, may be accompanied by anal chancre due to neighbouring autoinoculation [7].

In both sexes. Mixed chancre can be observed. It is due to the association with syphilis. The chancre is slightly indurated and not very painful. Extra-genital chancres have been described: herpetiform hand chancres, pelvic or abdominal localisations related to self-contamination and, exceptionally, oral or anal chancres [7, 9].

Complications. The spontaneous evolution is towards the multiplication of chancres and above all phagedenisms, with amputation of the penis. Treatment gives good results, with minimal sequelae such as indelible scars.

3. Diagnosis

A positive diagnosis is made when Ducrey's bacillus is found in the lesion. It is not usually found in lymph node puncture fluid. The diagnosis can be made by careful direct examination. Culture is difficult, as the germ does not grow easily on special media (Mueller Hilton chocolate gelose or enriched horse blood) after repeated sampling of the edges of the lesions. Molecular biology (PCR) has good sensitivity and specificity [10, 11].

In practice, the diagnosis of chancre mou is made in conjunction with other causes of genital ulceration, particularly those of sexually transmitted origin [10, 12].

- The syphilitic chancre is often a single, painless, dwarfed chancre.
- Herpes: multiple ulcerations in clusters, very superficial.
- The chancre of lymphogranulomatosis venereum or donovanosis.
- Rarely, it is necessary to discuss the great aphthosis or certain pyodermites.

4. Treatment

Ceftriaxone 250 mg intramuscularly (one dose) is particularly effective and is currently the treatment of choice for chancre mou [13].

Azithromycin 1g taken once orally is also highly effective. Erythromycin: 2g daily for 10 days [14].

Iterative punctures of the bubo contents are essential to relieve the patient.

References

1. Sehgal VN, Srivastava G. Chancroid: contemporary appraisal. Int J Dermatol 2003; 42 :182-90

2. Lewis DA, Mitja O. Haemophilus ducreyi: from sexually transmitted infection to skin pathogen. Cur Opin Infect Dis 2016 ; 19 :52-7
3. SteenR. Eradicating chancroid. Bull World Health Organ. 2001;79:818-26
4. Mungati M, Machiha A, Mugurungi O et al. The Etiology of Genital Ulcer Disease and Coinfections With Chlamydia trachomatis and Neisseria gonorrhoeae in Zimbabwe: Results From the Zimbabwe STI Etiology Study. Sex Transm Dis 2018;45:61-68.
5. DiCarlo RP, Martin DH. The clinical diagnosis of genital ulcer disease in men. Clin Infect Dis 1997 ;25 : 292-8
6. Mohammed TT, Olumide YM. Chancroid and human immunodeficiency virus infection: a review. Int J Dermatol 2008;47:1-8.
7. BendickC. Sexually Transmitted Infections in the Tropics. Hautarzt 2018;69:945-959.
8. Basta-Juzbasic A, Ceovic R. Chancroid, lymphogranuloma venereum, granuloma inguinale, genital herpes simplex infection, and molluscum contagiosum.Clin Dermatol. 2014;32:290-8.
9. Goens JL, Schwartz RA, De Wolf K. Mucocutaneous manifestations of chancroid, lymphogranuloma venereum and granuloma inguinale. Am Fam Physician1994;49: 415-8, 423-5.
10. Roett MA. Genital ulcers: differential diagnosis and management. Am Fam Physician. 2020 Mar 15;101(6):355-361.
11. Risbud A, Chan-Tack K, Gadkari D et al. The etiology of genital ulcer disease by multiplex polymerase chain reaction and relationship to HIV infection among patients attending sexually transmitted disease clinics in Pune, India. Sex Transm Dis 1999;26:55-62
12. Pitche P. Sexually transmitted ulcerations. EMC-Dermatologie 2022; 24 : 1-5 [article 98-450-A-10].
13. Centers for Diseases Control and Prevention. Sexually transmitted infections treatement. Guidelines 2021. MMR 2021; 70: 30-59
14. Romeo L ; Huerfano C, Grillo-Ardila CF. Macrolides for treatment of haemophilis ducreyi infection. Cochrane Database Sys Rev 2017; 12; CD012492

Venereal lymphogranulomatosis

1. Pathogen

First described in 1913, venereal lymphogranulomatosis (LGV) or Nicolas and Favre disease (named after the authors who described it) is an STI caused by 3 serotypes (L1, L_2 , L_3) of Chlamydia trachomatis [1]. A cosmopolitan disease, LGV is particularly common in tropical areas (South America, India, South-East Asia, sub-Saharan Africa) [2, 3]. Since the early 2000s, a resurgence of LGV has been observed in Europe and the United States among men who have sex with men [4-6].

2. Symptomatology

The signs are polymorphic and generally evolve in three stages.

Primary accident (chancre, proctitis)

After an average incubation period of 4 to 30 days, signs of the primary phase appear. The primary lesion is usually a small papule or vesicle which evolves into a painless, non-induced ulceration, usually healing within a few days without scarring [7-9]. This lesion corresponds to the point of inoculation of the germ.

In men, the chancre can be found on the glans or on the sheath; when it is intrameatic, the chancre manifests itself as a non-gonococcal urethral discharge. In women, the lesion may occur on the lips or on the vaginal wall. In men who have sex with men and women who have anal intercourse, there is an anorectal infection with a fairly noisy picture comprising a diarrhoeal syndrome, tenesmus and bloody, mucopurulent secretions [5, 6]. Histological examination may reveal diffuse inflammation with cryptic abscesses and giant cell granulomas. A particular feature of the clinical manifestations of LGV in men who have sex with men is the high frequency of rectitis or proctitis [10-13].

Secondary accident (inguinal adenitis).

Secondary manifestations are dominated by lymph node syndrome [6-8].

In men, lymph node involvement is mainly inguinal. It is generally multi-nodal. These are unilateral adenopathies consisting of several inflamed lymph nodes with periadenitis, giving the sign of lymph node disruption [9]. Involvement is unilateral in 60% of cases [2]. After several days, the skin around the adenopathy becomes inflamed, taut and violated. The affected lymph nodes coalesce to form an initially firm mass, which fluctuates later and forms an inguinal bubo. At this stage, and in the case of femoro-inguinal involvement, Poupart's inguinal ligament divides the mass into two lobules, giving the "pulley sign" characteristic of LGV [1, 2, 8]. Rarely, the bubo may heal spontaneously, but fistulisation of the skin is more common. Many fistulas leak pus (watering-can fistulas) and result in poroadenolymphitis.

In women, inguinal lymph node involvement may be observed. But inguinal adenitis is rare because of the lymphatic drainage of the female pelvic tract. Node involvement may be seen when the site of the primary lesion is the clitoris or a large lip. Rarely, deep lymph nodes may communicate with the digestive or genital tract, resulting in anal, recto-vaginal, recto-vesical and ischio-rectal fistulas [1, 5].

Tertiary stage

Complications are the result of untreated secondary lesions. These complications have become rare with the advent of effective antibiotics. However, even without treatment, only 10-20% of patients will develop these complications [7]. The manifestations of this stage include fibrous rectal stenosis. The rectal wall is thickened, rigid and severely ulcerated. The rectum may also be the site of vegetative rectitis with lobulated anal growths [14, 15]. LGV may be complicated by stricture of the urethra and elephantiasis of the external genitalia. In women, LGV can lead to esthiomene, with vesico-vaginal fistulas, vulvar elephantiasis and often rectal stricture. Anorectal and vulvar neoplastic degeneration is possible. Epidermoid carcinomas may graft onto LGV rectal stenoses.

3. Diagnosis

Positive diagnosis is based on the isolation of Chlamydia trachomatis L strains by culture (Mac Coy cell culture) and PCR (polymerase chain reaction) [13, 16]. Direct immunofluorescence is a diagnostic method other than culture and PCR. Serological diagnosis is based on the complement fixation reaction and the indirect immunofluorescence reaction. Other serological tests using the ELISA technique or radioimmunoassays are also highly sensitive but less specific [8]. Rectoscopy and histopathological examination of infected tissues (rectal mucosa, bubo) are non-specific [1].

Chancre should be discussed with other causes of sexually transmitted ulceration [17]. Inguinal adenopathies should be discussed with syphilis, chancroid mou, herpes, but also with gum tuberculosis, histoplasmosis and in some cases mycetoma and cat's claw disease [17]. Anorectal localisations may be confused with amoebiasis, Crohn's disease or any other pathology with an anorectal focus [17, 18].

4. Treatment

The treatment of choice is based on cyclins [18, 19]: tetracycline 2g per day for 2 to 4 weeks or doxycycline 200 mg per day for three weeks. Azithromycin is effective at a dose of 1g per week for 3 weeks [20].

In the event of complications, surgery is essential.

References

1. Collins L, White JA, Bradbeer C. Lymphogranuloma venereum. BMJ 2006;332:66. doi: 10.1136/bmj.332.7533.66.

2. Pitche P, Plinga A, Tchangai-Walla K. Lyphogranuloma venereum. Sante 1997;3:239-44

3. BendickC. Sexually Transmitted Infections in the Tropics. Hautarzt 2018;69:945-959

4. Ciccarese G, Drago F, Paradi A. Updates on lymphogranuloma venereum. J Eur Acad Dermatol Venereol 2021; 35: 1606-7

5. Nieuwenhuis RF, Bradley P Ossewaarde JM et al. Resurgence of lymphogranuloma venereum in Western Europe: an outbreak of Chlamydia trachomatis serovar l2 proctitis in The Netherlands among men who have sex with men. Clin Infect Dis 2004;39: 996-1003.
6. Kapoor S. Re-emergence of lymphogranuloma venereum. J Eur Acad Dermatol Venereol 2008 ;22:409-16.
7. White JA. Manifestations and management of lymphogranuloma venereum. Curr Opin Infect Dis. 2009;22: 57-66.
8. Caumes E, Dupin N, Janier M et al. Lymphogranuloma venereum. Ann Dermatol Venereol. 2016;143:736-738.
9. Stoner BP, Cohen SE. Lymphogranuloma Venereum: clinical presentation, diagnosis, and treatment. Clin Infect Dis 2015 ;61 Suppl 8:S865-73.
10. Richardson D, Goldmeier D. Lymphogranuloma venereum: an emerging cause of proctitis in men who have sex with men. Int J STD AIDS. 2007;18:11-4
11. Turner AN, Reese PC, Ervin M et al. HIV, rectal chlamydia, and rectal gonorrhea in men who have sex with men attending a sexually transmitted disease clinic in a midwestern US city. Sex Transm Dis 2013;40:433-8.
12. Hughes Y, Chen MY, Fairley CK et al. Universal lymphogranuloma venereum (LGV) testing of rectal chlamydia in men who have sex with men and detection of asymptomatic LGV. Sex Transm Infect. 2022;98:582-585
13. Dos Santos-Ferreira AC, Calanca R, Ardengh JC. Challenges in diagnosis of the ulcerative rectitis by Lymphogranuloma venereum in *Chlamydia trachomatis* infection and AIDS. Cureus 2023;15:e35420. doi: 10.7759/cureus.35420.
14. Ceovic R, Gulin SJ. Lymphogranuloma venereum: diagnostic and treatment challenges. Infect Drug Resist 2015;8:39-47
15. Kritikos A, Filippidis P. Lymphogranuloma venereum proctis. Sex Trans Dis 2021; 48 ; e33 doi/ 10.1097
16. Risbud A, Chan-Tack K, Gadkari D et al. The etiology of genital ulcer disease by multiplex polymerase chain reaction and relationship to HIV infection among patients attending sexually transmitted disease clinics in Pune, India. Sex Transm Dis 1999;26:55-62
17. Pitche P. Sexually transmitted ulcerations. EMC-Dermatologie 2022; 24 : 1-5 [article 98-450-A-10].
18. Roett MA. Genital ulcers: differential diagnosis and management. Am Fam Physician. 2020;101:355-361.
19. De Vries HJC, de Barbeyrac B, de Vrieze NHN et al. 2019 Eurpean guidelines on the management of lymphogranuloma venereum. J Eur Acad Dermatol 2019;33 :1821-28
20. Centers for Diseases Control and Prevention. Sexually transmitted infections treatement. Guidelines 2021. MMR 2021; 70: 30-59

Donovanose

1. Causal agent

Donovanosis (or granuloma inguinale) is a bacterial infection with sexual, inguinal, perineal and sometimes oral foci caused by *Klebsiella granulomatis* (formerly *Calymmatobacterium granulomatosis)* [1]. Donovanosis occurs mainly in tropical countries, particularly in south-east Asia, Latin America and the West Indies, central Australia, and central and southern Africa [2]. It is a highly non-contagious disease whose transmission requires multiple contacts between sexual partners in poor hygiene conditions. It is more common in men than in women [3].

2. Symptomatology

Incubation varies between 17 and 50 days [2, 3]. It begins as an indurated papule that softens, and the ulcer progresses. In the state phase, a polycyclic, rounded ulcerogranular placard with a sharp, often eversed border, bright red in colour, with a moist surface and a slightly fresher consistency, is present. The ulcerations may be multiple and coalesce to form a vast placard [4]. There is no satellite adenopathy. Lesions occur on the external genitalia, perineum and inguinal region. When there is intra- and subcutaneous spread from the penis or large lips, the disease spreads to the inguinal area in the form of ulcerating cellulitis known as "pseudobubo". Extension of the lesions can lead to disfigurement of the external genitalia [5].

Spontaneous evolution leads to complications: self-amputation of the external genitalia, infiltration of soft tissues, septicemia, cancerisation (epidermoid carcinoma). It should be noted that septicemia (or disseminated donovanosis) occurs mainly in women, in whom the chancre goes unnoticed. Dissemination, which is fairly rare, gives rise to metastatic systemic infections, predominantly of the bone (bone and joint involvement in multiple sites), liver and lungs [4, 5].

In endemic areas, the association of donovanosis with syphilis, herpes and HIV infection is relatively frequent. Any patient presenting with donovanosis or genital ulceration should therefore be tested for HIV.

3. Diagnosis

Diagnostic confirmation is based on the presence of Donovan bodies on a smear by direct examination of ulcero-vegetative lesions, or by biopsy, which reveals Donovan bodies within mononucleated cells [5]. There are no serological tests available for the diagnosis of Donovanosis. *Klebsiella granulomatis* has recently been cultured in monocytes (specialised laboratories). PCR and serology are not commonly used [6].

In the presence of genital ulceration, it is important to consider other ulcerative diseases with a genital focus: syphilis, herpes, chancroid, lymphogranulomatosis, schistosomiasis, cutaneous amoebiasis and ulcero-vegetative carcinoma [7, 8].

4. Treatment

Many antibiotics are effective [9, 10]. Streptomycin: 2 grams morning and evening for 5 days or 1g a day for 15 days. Ceftriaxone: 2g a day for 4 days. Cyclines: tetracycline 2g a day (or doxycycline 200mg a day) for 15 days. Azithromycin 1g/week for 4 weeks.

References

1. Richens J. Donovanosis Sex Transm Infect 2006; 82 (suppl 4): 22-25
2. Belda Junior W. Donovanosis. An Bras Dermatol 2020; 95: 67-83
3. Causes E, Janier M, Dupin N et al. Donovanosis. Ann Dermatol Venereol 2016; 143: 72940
4. Richens J. Donovanosis (granuloma inguinale). Sex Transm Infect 2006;82(Suppl 4):iv21-2.
5. O'Farrell N. Clinico-epidemiological study of donovanosis in Durban, South Africa. Genitourin Med1993;69:108-11.
6. Muller EE, Kularatne R. The changing epidemiology of genital ulcer disease in South Africa: has donovanosis been eliminated? Sex Transm Infect 2020; 96:596-600.
7. Ahmed N, Pillay A, Lawler M et al. Donovanosis causing lymphadenitis, mastoiditis, and meningitis in a child. Lancet 2015; 385:2644.
8. Pitche P. Sexually transmitted ulcerations. EMC-Dermatologie 2022; 24 : 1-5 [article 98-450-A-10].
9. O'Farrell N, Hoosen A, Kingston M. 2018 UK national guideline for the management of donovanosis. Int J STD AIDS 2018;29:946-948.
10. Centers for Diseases Control and Prevention. Sexually transmitted infections treatement. Guidelines 2021. MMR 2021; 70: 30-59

Table 6: Etiological work-up for genital ulceration [8].

Ulceration aгдuë (< 1 month)	Culture and/or PCR: HSV2, HSV 1 Darkfield microscope or PCR, Syphilis serology HIV serology Direct examination: for Haemophilus ducreyi and Donovan bodies, PCR after detection of H. *ducreyi* by culture

	PCR *Chlamydia trachomatis*
Chronic ulceration (>1 month)	Culture and/or PCR: HSV2, HSV 1 HSV2 specific serology, HSV1 if PCR and culture negative (recurrent herpes) HIV and syphilis serologies

PART IV

IV. OTHER SEXUALLY TRANSMITTED INFECTIONS **Other sexually transmitted infections**

Human papillomavirus genital infections

1. Causal agent

HPVs belong to the Papovavirus family *(Papovaviridae'),* which are all DNA viruses. There are 5 main HPV genera (*alpha, beta, gamma, mu, nu*) with at least 60% genomic homology [1]. Condylomas are caused by genital infection with the *human papillomavirus (HPV).* There are several serotypes of HPV, but only a few can be sexually transmitted: types 6 and 11 for ano-genital condylomas; types 16, 18, 31 or 33 for cervical dysplasia [1-3]. The major risk of condyloma or genital HPV infection is the risk of induction of genital cancers [3-6].

Various studies indicate that the prevalence and incidence of genital papilloma virus infections have increased considerably in recent years [7]. In fact, these conditions are one of the main reasons for consultations at STD clinics. There are many asymptomatic carriers, particularly women [4-6]. The median time taken for condylomata to develop in men after infecting contact is 17 months [6]. Transmission from mother to child (*in utero* or often during childbirth) is possible.

2. Symptomatology

In men

Condylomata acuminata and exophytica. These are soft, fleshy, vegetative tumours whose preferred sites are the frenulum, the balano-preputial fold and the prepuce [8-10]. In humid areas, they take on giant forms. Localisation in the urethra may cause urethral discharge, genes during micturition and bleeding with or without haematuria. Perianal sites are more sensitive and vegetative.

*Flat condyloma***.** These are pigmented papules usually found on the cutaneous surface of the penis, penis and anal margin, particularly in men who have sex with men [8].

Subclinical condylomatous lesions. They are classically on the cutaneous side and are revealed by acetic acid. On the meat and distal urethra (at the penis), they appear as punctate lesions. On the mucous membranes, these condylomas appear as whitish macules [9].

In women

There are also condylomata acuminata on the fork and small yeast, and exophytic condylomata typical of the cervix, which can crack, macerate and become infected, causing pain and discomfort. Flat condylomas of the cervix are more difficult to diagnose [11]. The majority of flat condylomata of the uterus are clinically invisible in the naked eye. The application of acetic acid enables them to be visualised. Colposcopy reveals whitish spots or a simple epithelial stain, hence the importance of systematic cervical cancer screening, which is recommended for all women with one or more risk factors. In fact, the real problem posed by HPV infection in women is the close association between condylomas (often subclinical) and cervical dysplasia: it should be emphasised that HPV infection is the leading cause of cervical cancer [3].

Condylomatous lesions without cellular atypia regress on average in 30-40% of cases, persist in 50% of cases and progress in 7-10% of cases [3]. Lesion progression is correlated with cellular atypia and the degree of cervical dysplasia. Progression is also correlated with viral type. Depending on the risk of oncogenicity, HPVs are classified as low risk (6, 11, 40, 42, 43, 44), intermediate risk (26, 55, 66, 67, 70, 73, 82) and high risk (16, 18, 32, 33, 35, 39, 45, 51, 52, 56, 58; 59; 60) [2]. The risk of degeneration of cervical dysplasia in women should encourage all practitioners to systematically offer cervico-vaginal smears to the partners of men with condyloma.

In both sexes: giant condylomas (Bushke-Lowenstein tumour) can be observed. These are vegetative tumours several centimetres in diameter, sometimes infiltrating [6, 11]. These tumours often occur on the lips and perineal area in women, or in the ano-genital area. This type of condyloma can rapidly degenerate into a carcinoma. Sometimes, when these lesions are highly infiltrative with a mucosal preponderance, histologically they are already carcinoma in situ [3].
In children, the presence of anogenital warts raises the issue of possible sexual abuse [12-14]. Depending on the age of the child and the findings of the clinical examination, all possible routes of non-sexual transmission (mother-child, contact with warts in the family) and sexual transmission (possible sexual abuse) should be investigated, with the resulting medical and legal implications. In fact, in 3 to 30% of cases, a notion of sexual abuse is found [12, 14].

3. Diagnosis

Clinically, it is easy to remove visible lesions. Application of acetic acid can help visualise flat condylomas [2, 4]. In women, the application of acetic acid to the cervix enables the diagnosis to be made during a routine gynaecological examination.

Diagnosis of certainty is based on detection of HPV by electron microscopy, detection of the capsidal antigen by immunohistochemistry, detection of viral DNA by molecular hybridisation, or genomic amplification of viral sequences by PCR [15]. These different techniques are the responsibility of specialist laboratories.

In countries with limited resources, histology is a good diagnostic guide [10]: it shows elongated dermal papillae, hyperplasia of the *stratum spinosum* with hyperkeratosis, and vacuolated cells with irregular hyperchromatic nuclei (koilocytes) containing viral particles. Peniscopy and colonoscopy can be used to visualise mucosal lesions and possibly take a biopsy. The advantage of histology is that it can detect incipient dysplasia or neoplasia that is already present.

Condylomata acuminata rarely pose a differential diagnostic problem. Molluscum, overload disease (mucinosis, xanthomas), botriomyomata and genital mucosal plaques of secondary syphilis must be ruled out. Flat condylomas may be mistaken for simple post-inflammatory leukomelanodermal spots [8].

4.Treatment

Cryotherapy or the application of podophyllin resin (1-2 times a week) is a good treatment for localised, non-bulky condylomata [10, 16-18]. Electrocautery and cryosurgery are also highly effective in multiple and large condylomas. The CO $laser_2$ is indicated for cervical condylomas [16]. Immunomodulatory treatments such as imiquimod and interferon are also used with varying degrees of success, particularly for recurrent or multiple condylomas [16]. Vaccination against HPV infection is highly effective in reducing the incidence of condyloma and, above all, in preventing cervical cancer [19, 20].

References

1. Weaver BA. Epidemiology and natural history of genital human papillomavirus infection.J Am Osteopath Assoc 2006;106 (3 Suppl 1):S2-8.

2. Bouvard V, Baan R, Straif K et al. A review of human carcinogens; Part B: biological agents. Lancet Oncol 2009;10:321-2. doi: 10.1016/s1470-2045(09)70096-8.

3. Chelimo C, Wouldes TA, Cameron LD et al. Risk factors for and prevention of human papillomaviruses (HPV), genital warts and cervical cancer. J Infect 2013; 66:207-17

4. De Vuyst H, Alemany L, Lacey C et al. The burden of human papillomavirus infections and related diseases in sub-Saharan Africa. Vaccine 2013; 31 (Suppl 5):F32-46.

5. Lekoane KMB, Kuupiel D, Mashamba-Thompson TP et al. Evidence on the prevalence, incidence, mortality and trends of human papilloma virus-associated cancers in sub-Saharan Africa: systematic scoping review. BMC Cancer 2019;19:563. doi: 10.1186/s12885-019-5781- 3.

6. Banura C, Mirembe FM, Orem J et al. Prevalence, incidence and risk factors for anogenital warts in Sub Saharan Africa: a systematic review and meta analysis. Infect Agent Cancer

2013;8:27. doi: 10.1186/1750-9378-8-27.

7. Tyros G, Mastraftsi S, Gregoriou S. Incidence of anogenital warts: epidemiological risk factors and real-life impact of human papillomavirus vaccination. Int J STD AIDS 2021;32:4- 13.

8. von Krogh G, G Gross G. Anogenital warts. Clin Dermatol1997;15:355-68.

9. Obalek S, Jablonska S, G Orth G.Anogenital warts in children. Clin Dermatol 1997;15:369-76.

10. Anoukoum T, Baeta S, Attipou K et al. Venereal vegetations of the urogenital tract and their urological complications. Apropos of 257 cases. J Urol (Paris). 1996;102:212-5.

11. Santos FLSG, Inven^ao MCV, Araujo ED et al. Comparative analysis of different PCR-based strategies for HPV detection and genotyping from cervical samples. J Med Virol. 2021; 93:6347-6354.

12. Rogstad KE, Wilkinson D, Robinson A. Sexually transmitted infections in children as a marker of child sexual abuse and direction of future research. Curr Opin Infect Dis 2016; 29:414.

13. Pitche P, Kombate K, Gbadoe AD et al. Sexually transmitted diseases in young children in Lome (Togo). Role of sexual abuse. Arch Pediatr 2001; 8:25-31

14. Awasthi S, Ornelas J, Armstrong A et al. Anogenital warts and relationship to child sexual abuse: Systematic review and meta-analysis. Pediatr Dermatol 2021; 38:842-850.

15. Partridge JM, Hughes JP, Feng Q, et al. Genital human papillomavirus infection in men: incidence and risk factors in a cohort of university students. J Infect Dis 2007;196:1128-36.

16. Ntanasis-Stathopoulos I, Kyriazoglou A, Liontos M et al. Current trends in the management and prevention of human papillomavirus (HPV) infection. J BUON 2020; 25:1281-1285.

17. Bertolotti A, Dupin N, Bouscarat F, et al. Cryotherapy to treat anogenital warts in nonimmunocompromised adults: Systematic review and meta-analysis. J Am Acad Dermatol. 2017;7e:518-526.

18. Centers for Diseases Control and Prevention. Sexually transmitted infections treatement. Guidelines 2021. MMR 2021; 70: 30-59

19. Nofa A, Al-Shimaa M, Ibrahim M et al. Human papillomavirus and vaccination J Am Acad Dermatol2023 ;88:e177. doi: 10.1016/j.jaad.2020.05.004.

20. Mariani L, Preti M, Cristoforoni P et al. Overview of the benefits and potential issues of the nonavalent HPV vaccine. Int J Gynaecol Obstet 2017;136:258-265.

HIV infection

1. Causal agent

Human immunodeficiency viruses (HIV) belong to the retrovirus family. The retrovirus family is classified according to morphological, phylogênic or pathogênic criteria into three subfamilies [1, 2]. *i)* RNA oncoviruses: these are often associated with leukaemia (HTLV: Huma T-Cell Leukemia virus) and four subtypes are known (HTLV- 1 and HTLV-2, HTLV-3, HTLV-4). ii) Lentiviruses are viruses that cause slowly progressing diseases (pneumonia, neurological disorders) and are cytopathogenic in culture. iii) Human immunodeficiency viruses (HIV 1 and HIV 2). HIV 1 is the most widespread virus in the world, on every continent, and is responsible for the majority of cases of infection. HIV 2 is described specifically in West Africa. HIV is transmitted by sex, blood and from mother to child. Over the past 40 years, HIV infection has become a major public health problem, with more than 39 million deaths [3].

The natural history of HIV infection helps us to understand the richness of the symptomatology, which varies according to the degree of immunodepression [4].

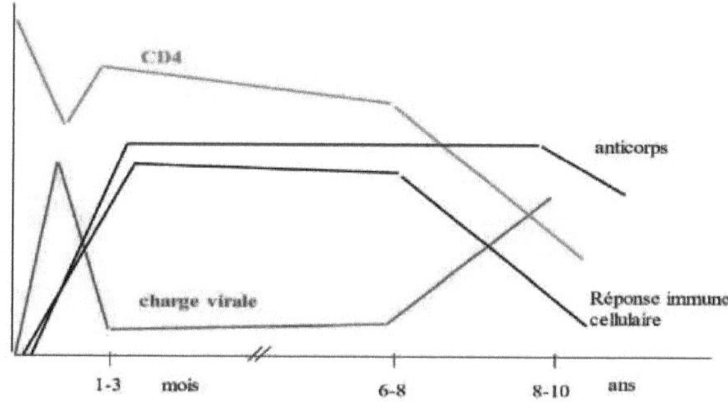

Figure 6: Natural history of HIV infection [1].

2. Symptomatology

HIV infection is characterised by a high degree of clinical polymorphism due to the wide range of organs affected by opportunistic infections, the frequency and severity of which increase with the level of immunodepression [5]. Over the last twenty years or so, all countries have made significant progress in the fight against this pandemic, leading to widespread access to antiretroviral treatment for people living with HIV. As a result, we have seen fewer and fewer cases of AIDS in clinical practice in recent years, compared with the peak of the pandemic in the 1980s and 1990s.

Primary infection

The clinical manifestations of HIV infection at this stage are non-specific and highly variable. The first symptoms often appear between 10 and 15 days. Slightly more than half of infected subjects are considered to have clinical manifestations between two and six weeks [5-7]. The signs are dominated by an influenza-like syndrome with fever, myalgias, headache, dysphagia and sometimes asthenia [7]. The clinical signs that should attract attention are maculopapular exanthema and superficial adenopathy. The exanthema affects the trunk and sometimes the face. This exanthema may be associated with oral ulcerations. In addition to cutaneous signs, superficial adenopathy may appear during the second week. These are multiple adenopathies: axillary, cervical and inguinal. These adenopathies regress slowly over several weeks or months. Gastrointestinal symptoms are fairly rare and take the form of diarrhoea, sometimes associated with abdominal pain. Neurological manifestations such as meningoencephalitis and facial paralysis have been reported in 10% of cases. However, several scientific studies have shown that almost 70% of people infected at this stage do not present any symptoms, hence the importance of an active screening strategy for anyone behaving at risk [8].

Table 7: Frequency of clinical and laboratory signs in symptomatic patients at the time of primary HIV infection [7].

Symptoms	**Frequency (%)**
Fever	> 90
Weight loss	15-50
Pharyngitis	40-77
Maculopapular exanthema	53-73
Oral and/or genital ulcers	30-40
Polyadenopathy	57

Myalgia, arthralgia	30-60
Diarrhoea, nausea	33
Cephalees	29-55
Other neurological signs	13
Thrombocytopenia (< 1500)	74
Neutropenia	35
Anemie	26
Lymphopenia (< 1000)	30
Hepatic cytolysis	23-46

Manifestations other than primary infection

After the primary infection stage, the main clinical signs will appear as the immune system becomes depressed, following the natural history of HIV infection. Indeed, the majority of signs associated with opportunistic infections and diseases appear throughout the natural history of HIV infection, particularly at the AIDS stage [1, 2].

All organs are affected by the different types of opportunistic disease (infectious, tumour, inflammatory). The organs most affected by HIV infection are the lungs, digestive tract, skin and nervous system [1, 2, 9-13] (Table).

Table 8: Main clinical manifestations of HIV infection by organ

Organs	**Conditions**
Lungs	• Tuberculosis, pyogenes pneumonia • Pneumocystis, cryptococcosis, histoplasmosis, aspergillosis • Toxoplasmosis • Cytomegalovirus (CMV) pneumonia. • Bronchial cancers, Kaposi's disease, haemopathies • Sarcoidosis, lymphoid interstitial lung disease
Nervous system	*Damage to the central nervous system* • Toxoplasmosis, cryptococcosis, CMV encephalitis, syphilis • Progressive multiple leukoencephalitis, stroke *Peripheral involvement* - symmetrical distal polyneuropathy
Skin	• Varicella zoster, mucocutaneous herpes, oral hairy leukoplakia (EBV), HPV infection • Folliculitis, ecthyma furuncles, bacterial dermohypodermatitis, bacillary angiomatosis, syphilis • Candidiasis, dermatophytes, histoplasmosis, cryptococcosis, penicilinosis, molluscum contagiosum • Leishmaniasis, scabiosis • Kaposi's disease, squamous cell carcinoma • Prurigo, seborrheic dermatitis, psoriasis, xerosis, eczema, toxidermia • Hair abnormalities (canitis, spontaneous hair loss or silky trichopathy in black people)
Digestive tract	• Oesophageal candidiasis, infectious diarrhoea, • Non-infectious diarrhoea, tumours (lymphoma, Kaposi's disease, adenocarcinoma) • Viral hepatitis and carcinoma
Eyes	• CMV retinitis, herpetic necrotizing retinopathy • Eye disease (syphilis, cryptococcosis, tuberculosis, pneumocystis)

Hematopoietic system	• Lymphomas (Burkitt's lymphoma, HHV8-associated lymphomas, EBV-associated lymphoblastic lymphomas) • Hodgkin's lymphoma, primary cerebral lymphoma • Castelman's disease • Cytopenias (thrombocytopenic purpura, autoimmune anemia)

3. Classification of HIV and AIDS

Given the symptomatic (clinical and biological) polymorphism of HIV infection and the non-specific nature of the signs, classifications were proposed at the start of this epidemic by the World Health Organisation (WHO) and the Center of Diseases Control in Atlanta (CDC) [14, 15]. These classifications have a dual diagnostic and prognostic function, and have long been used to define therapeutic strategies and monitor patients.

While the CDC classification is the one most used in developed countries, the WHO classification is the most appropriate for resource-limited countries when it comes to managing PLHIV, and has been regularly updated (the latest WHO classification dates from 2007).

Table 9: CDC classification of HIV infection for adults and adolescents (1993)

	Clinical categories		
Number of lymphocytes	A Asymptomatic Primary infection Persistent generalized lymphadenopathy	B Symptomatic Without A or C criteria	C AIDS
> 500/mm3	Al	Bl	C1
200-499/mm32	A2	B2	C2
< 200/mm3	A3	B3	C3

*Note: * The clinical categories are described in the CDC clinical classification table below.*

Table 10: CDC 1993 classification for adults and adolescents (clinical categories)

Category A

One or more of the criteria listed below in an HIV-infected adult or adolescent, if there are no criteria in categories B and C :

- Asymptomatic HIV infection
- Persistent generalized lymphadenopathy
- Symptomatic primary infection

Category B

Clinical manifestations in an HIV-infected adult or adolescent that do not fall into the following category C and which meet at least one of the following conditions:

- Bacillary angiomatosis
- Oropharyngeal andidosis
- Persistent, frequent vaginal andidosis or poor response to treatment
- Cervical dysplasia (moderate or severe), carcinoma in situ
- Constitutional syndrome: fever (38°5 C) or diarrhoea lasting more than 1 month
- Hairy tongue leukoplakia
- Recurrent shingles or shingles invading more than one dermatome
- Idiopathic thrombocytopenic purpura
- Listeriosis
- Peripheral neuropathy

Category C

This category corresponds to the definition of AIDS in adults. When a subject has presented one of the pathologies on this list, he or she is definitively classified in category C:

- Bronchial, tracheal or extrapulmonary andidosis
- C andidosis of the oesophagus
- Invasive cervical cancer
- Disseminated or extrapulmonary coccidioidomycosis
- Extrapulmonary cryptococcosis
- Intestinal cryptosporidiosis evolving for more than a month

- CMV infection (other than liver, spleen or lymph nodes)
- CMV Retinitis
- Encephalopathy due to HIV
- Herpetic infection, chronic ulcers lasting more than 1 month; or bronchial, pulmonary or oesophageal infection
- Disseminated or extrapulmonary histoplasmosis
- Chronic intestinal isosporidiosis (more than one month)
- Kaposi's sarcoma
- Burkitt's lymphoma
- Immunoblastic lymphoma
- Primary cerebral lymphoma
- Infection with Mycobacterium tuberculosis, regardless of location (pulmonary or extrapulmonary)
- Infection with identified or unidentified mycobacteria, disseminated or extrapulmonary
- Pneumonic a pneumocystis carinii
- Recurrent bacterial pneumonia
- Progressive multifocal leukoencephalitis
- Septicemic a salmonella non typhi recurrente
- HIV-related cachectic syndrome
- Cerebral toxoplasmosis

Table 11: WHO classification of clinical stages

Clinical stage I

- Asymptomatic patient.
- Persistent generalized adenopathy accompanied by fever.

Clinical stage II

- Weight loss of less than 10% of body weight.
- Minor mucocutaneous manifestations (seborrheic dermatitis, prurigo, onychomycosis, recurrent mouth ulcers, angular cheilitis).
- Herpetic infection (shingles...) in the last five years.
- Recurrent upper respiratory tract infections (bacterial sinusitis).

Clinical stage III

- Super weight loss! 10% of body weight.
- Chronic unexplained diarrhoea for more than a month.
- Prolonged unexplained fever for over a month.
- Oral thrush.
- Oral hairy leukoplakia.
- Pulmonary tuberculosis in previous farmee.
- Severe bacterial infections (e.g. pneumonia).
- Acute necrotizing ulcerative stomatitis
- Persistent anaemia (haemoglobin <8g/dl)
- Neutropenia (<500/mm3)
- Chronic thrombocytopenia (platelet count < 50,000/mm3)

Clinical stage IV

- AIDS cachectic syndrome
- Pneumocystis.
- Cerebral toxoplasmosis.
- Cryptosporidiosis with diarrhoea > 1 month.
- Chronic intestinal isosporosis (> 1 month)
- Extrapulmonary cryptococcosis.
- Chronic cutaneous-mucosal *herpes simplex* (lasting more than one month) or visceral *herpes simplex* (of any duration)
- Cytomegalovirus with organ involvement other than liver, spleen or lymph nodes.
- Herpetic infection, mucocutaneous infection > 1 month, or visceral infection of any duration.
- Progressive multifocal leukoencephalopathy.
- Any generalized endemic mycosis (such as histoplasmosis, coccidioidomycosis).
- Candidiasis of the resophagus, trachea, branches or lungs.
- Generalized atypical mycobacteriosis.
- Non-typhoidal Salmonella septicemia.
- Extrapulmonary tuberculosis.

- Lymphoma (primary cerebral or non-Hodgkin's).
- Kaposi's sarcoma.
- Invasive cervical carcinoma
- Atypical disseminated leishmaniasis
- American reactive trypanosomiasis (meninencephalitis or myocarditis)
- Symptomatic nephropathy associated with HIV
- HIV encephalopathy

4. Diagnosis

Positive diagnosis of HIV infection is made using screening tests (serology) and molecular biology. High-performance screening tests (highly sensitive and highly specific) have been available for several years now. These include enzyme-linked immunosorbent assays (Elisa, immunoblot) [16-18]. These tests can also distinguish between HIV-1 and HIV-2.

Virological diagnosis using molecular biology enables qualitative tests (RNA PCR, HIV-1 DNA, ARV HIV-2 DNA PCR) to be carried out, as well as quantitative tests using viral load assays [19, 20].

5. Treatment

The treatment of HIV infection has been revolutionised by antiretroviral drugs, whose effective therapeutic combinations have considerably reduced AIDS-related mortality. Since the early 2000s, there has been a gradual harmonisation of strategies and recommendations for the treatment of PLHIV worldwide [3, 21-24]. In practice, the management of HIV involves both treatment of HIV with antiretroviral drugs and etiological treatment of opportunistic infections where appropriate.

Table 12: The main antiretroviral drugs [2].

) nucleoside reverse transcriptase inhibitors (INTRI)

ZidovudineAbacavirZalcitabine

Lamivudine, EmticitabineStavudine

Tenofovir alafenamide Tenofovir disoproxil fumarate Didanosine

Non-nucleoside reverse transcriptase inhibitors (NNRTIs).*

NevirapineEfavirenzEtravirine

RilprivirineDoravirine

Protease inhibitors (PIs)

Atazanavir	Lopinavir	Ritonavir
Daruvanir	Cobicistat	Saquinavir
Integrase (II) inhibitors		
Bictegravir	Cabotegravir	Doruvanir
Elvitegravir	Raltegravir	

CCR5 inhibitors

Maraviroc

*Note: * In general, non-nucleoside reverse transcriptase inhibitors are not effective against HIV-2.*

Therapeutic strategies

Therapeutic strategies are based on antiretroviral tritherapy combining, as first-line treatment, two nucleoside reverse transcriptase inhibitors (INTRI) with either a non-nucleoside reverse transcriptase inhibitor (NNRTI), a protease inhibitor (PI) or an integrase inhibitor (II) [21-25].

Outside the first line, second- and third-line regimens are more varied and depend on the problems of failure and resistance of first-line molecules [26-29]. Therapeutic regimens are regularly revised in all countries (European, American and WHO recommendations) in order to take into account changes in the level of resistance on the one hand, and scientific evidence concerning therapeutic lines and new molecules on the market on the other.

Management of opportunistic infections

In addition to treatment for HIV infection with ARVs, other treatments involve the management of opportunistic diseases (pulmonary, digestive, neurological, cutaneous and mucosal in particular).

Reference

1. Girard PM, Katlama C, Pialoux G. VIH. Edition 2011, Editions Doin, 2011

2. Katlama C, Ghosn J, Wandeler G. VIH, hepaties virales et sante sexuelle. Editions EDP Science Paris 2020

3. UNAIDS. Annual report 2022. www.unaids/annuel report 2022

4. Baggaley R, Dalal S, Johnson C et al. Beyond the 90-90-90: refocusing HIV prevention as part of the global HIV response.J Int AIDS Soc 2016;19:21348. doi: 0.7448/IAS.19.1.21348.

5. Sabin CA, Lundgren JD. The natural history of HIV infection. Curr Opin HIV AIDS 2013 ;8:311-7.

6. Stekler J, Collier AC. Primary HIV Infection. Curr HIV/AIDS Rep 2004 ;1:68-73

7. Cohen MS, Shaw GM, McMichael AJ et al. Acute HIV-1 infection. N Engl J Med 2011; 364 :1964-54

8. Cohen MS, Gay CL, Busch MP et al. The detection of acute HIV infection. J Infect Dis 2010; 202 (Suppl 2):S270-7

9. Umoru D, Oviawe O, Ibadin M et al. Mucocutaneous manifestation of pediatric human immunodeficiency virus/acquired immunodeficiency syndrome (HIV/AIDS) in relation to degree of immunosuppression: a study of a West African population. Int J Dermatol 2012;51:305-12

10. Pitche P, Tchangai-Walla K, Napo-Koura G et al. Prevalence of skin manifestations in AIDS patients in the Lome-Tokoin University Hospital (Togo). Sante 1995; 5:349-52.

11. Franquet T, Domingo P. Pulmonary Infections in People Living with HIV. Radiol Clin North Am 2022; 60:507-520

12. Eggers C, Arendt G, Hahn K et al. HIV-1-associated neurocognitive disorder: epidemiology, pathogenesis, diagnosis, and treatment. J Neurol 2017; 264:1715-1727.

13. Chang AY, Doiron P, Maurer T. Cutaneous malignancies in HIV. Curr Opin HIV AIDS. 2017;12:57-62

14. Center of Diseases Control and Prevention. CDC revises HIV classification system, AIDS definition. W V Med J1993;89:74.

15. World Health Organization. Interim WHO clinical staging of HIV/AIDS and HIV/AIDS case definitions for surveillance: Switzerland: World Health Organization; 2005.

16. Okusanya B, Kimaru LJ, Mantina N et al. Interventions to increase early infant diagnosis of HIV infection: A systematic review and meta-analysis. PLoS One 2022;17:e0258863. doi: 10.1371/journal.pone.0258863. eCollection 2022.

17. Alexander TS. Human Immunodeficiency Virus diagnostic testing: 30 years of evolution. Clin Vaccine Immunol 2016; 23:249-53.

18. Kusagawa S, Kawana-Tachikawa A, Matsubayashi K et al. Evaluation of Geenius HIV-1/2 Confirmatory Assay for the confirmatory and differential diagnosis of HIV-1/HIV-2 in Japan and reliability of the Geenius Reader in the diagnosis of HIV-2. BMC Infect Dis 2021;21:569. doi: 10.1186/s12879-021-06291-5.

19. Ochodo EA, Guleid F, Deeks JJ et al. Point-of-care tests detecting HIV nucleic acids for diagnosis of HIV-1 or HIV-2 infection in infants and children aged 18 months or less. Cochrane Database Syst Rev 2021; 8:CD013207. doi: 10.1002/14651858.CD013207

20. Anderson EM, Maldarelli F. Quantification of HIV DNA using droplet digital PCR techniques. Curr Protoc Microbiol 2018;5:e62. doi: 10.1002/cpmc.62.

21. Gandhi RT, Bedimo R, Hoy JF et al. Antiretroviral drugs for treatment and prevention of HIV infection in adults: 2022 Recommendations of the International Antiviral Society-USA Panel. JAMA 2023;329:63-84.

22. Wen Y, Bar KJ, Li JZ. Lessons learned from HIV antiretroviral treatment interruption trials. Curr Opin HIV AIDS 2018;13 :416-421.

23. Taylor BS, Tieu HO, Jones J et al. ROI 2019: advances in antiretroviral therapy.Top Antivir

Med 2019; 27:50-68.
24. Palich R. Current treatment of HIV infection. Rev Prat 2021;71:976-982.
25. Waters L, Winston A, Reeves I et al. BHIVA guidelines on antiretroviral treatment for adults living with HIV-1 2022. HIV Med 2022; 23 (Suppl 5):3-115.
26. Dagnra AY, Vidal N, Mensah A et al. High prevalence of HIV-1 drug resistance among patients on first-line antiretroviral treatment in Lome, Togo. J Int AIDS Soc 2011;14:30. doi: 10.1186/1758-2652-14-30.
27. L, Zhukova A, Villabona-Arenas CJet al. Drug resistance mutations in HIV: new bioinformatics approaches and challenges. Curr Opin Virol 2021;51:56-64.
28. Ji H, Patterson A, Taylor T et al. Prevalence of Primary Drug Resistance Against HIV-1 Integrase Inhibitors in Canada. J Acquir Immune Defic Syndr 2018;78:e1-e3. doi: 10.1097
29. Moreno M, Caballero E, Mateus RM et al. HIV drug resistance in Africa: an emerging problem that deserves urgent attention. JAIDS. 2017;31:1637-1639. doi: 10.1097

Viral hepatitis

1. Causal agent

There are four different viral hepatitis viruses: hepatitis A virus (HAV), hepatitis B virus (HBV), hepatitis C virus (HCV) and hepatitis delta. Hepatitis A is classically transmitted orally, usually in children, but it is also transmitted sexually through mouth-to-anal contact (feco-oral transmission) in men who have sex with men [1, 2]. In developed countries, where the incidence of this infection is low, there have been documented outbreaks and clusters of hepatitis A infection in 2015 and 2016 in Europe and the USA [2-3].

Evidence of sexual transmission of hepatitis B and C has been available for several years [1, 4, 5]. The HBS antigen has been demonstrated in blood and semen, saliva and vaginal secretions. This transmission is observed in both homosexuals and heterosexuals (cases of fulminant acute hepatitis have been reported in female partners of men with chronic hepatitis B) [6]. Sexual transmission of hepatitis C has been reported to be low in MSM and HIV-infected men [7-10].

2. Symptomatology

The clinical presentation of hepatitis A is generally uncommon (or even asymptomatic in most cases). Anorexia and fever precede the icteric phase. The disease progresses spontaneously, resolving with complete recovery within one to two months [1, 2].

Most cases of hepatitis B are asymptomatic. After a fairly long incubation period of 1 to 6 months following the onset of anicteric signs (headache, arthralgia, urticaria, fever, digestive disorders) [12]. The course is generally benign in the form of chronic carriage. Rarely, severe acute fulminant forms may be observed. The major problem with hepatitis B infections is chronic carriage, during which the patient may be contagious, and some chronic forms progress to cirrhosis and cancer [12-14]. Chronic, asymptomatic progression is characteristic of viral hepatitis C, which can lead to cancer.

3. Diagnosis

Viral hepatitis is diagnosed on the basis of markers (antigens and antibodies) in the case of hepatitis A, B and C [1, 13].

Enzyme-linked immunosorbent assays are currently very effective in diagnosing and screening for viral hepatitis. PCR is highly specific and is commonly used for diagnosis in developing countries [13].

4. Treatment

Antiviral drugs that are effective in treating hepatitis B and C have been available for around ten years. Indications for treatment are based on consensus criteria [13, 14, 15-20]. Treatment of viral hepatitis B is based on nucleoside analogues (entecabir) or nucleotide analogues (tenofovir disoproxil or tenofovir aleferamide) for 48 weeks. The indications and therapeutic regimens depend on the severity of the infection and must be adapted to the patient's clinical situation.

Given the frequent association of hepatitis B with HIV infection, the therapeutic lines comprising tenofovir and lamuvidine are the most appropriate for the management of people suffering from this co-infection. Unlike hepatitis C, there is currently no hope of curing hepatitis B, regardless of the drugs used. Treatment of hepatitis C is determined by genotyping (1 or 2).
Genotype 1 (the most frequent) is treated very effectively with the combination of sofosbuvir and velpatasvir or sofosbuvir and ledispasvir. These drugs cause high rates of warion in patients infected with hepatitis C.

References

1. Pinto RM, Perez-Rodriguez FJ, Costafreda MI, et al. Pathogenicity and virulence of hepatitis A virus. Virulence 2021;12:1174-1185.

2. Zhang XS, Ong JJ, Macgregor L, Vilaplana TG et al. Transmission dynamics of the 2016-18 outbreak of hepatitis A among men who have sex with men in England and cost-effectiveness analysis of vaccination strategies to prevent future outbreaks. Lancet Reg Health Eur 2022;19:100426. doi: 10.1016

3. Martin A, Meddeb L, Lagier JC et al. Hepatitis A outbreak in HIV-infected patients in Southeastern France: questions and responses? Epidemiol Infect 2020; 148:e79.doi: 10.1017/S0950268820000345.

4. Davis LG, Weber DJ, Lemon SM. Horizontal transmission of hepatitis B virus. Lancet 1989; 1:889-93

5. Brettler DB, Mannucci PM, Gringeri A et al. The low risk of hepatitis C transmission among sexual partners of hepatitis C-infected hemophilic males: an international multcenter study? Blood 1992; 80; 540-3

6. Lloyd AR, Franco RA. Sexual Transmission of Viral Hepatitis. Infect Dis Clin North Am 2023;37:335-349.

7. Brook MG. Sexually acquired hepatitis. Sex Transm Infect. 2002;78:235-40.

8. Bradshaw D, Vasylyeva TI, Davis C et al. Transmission of hepatitis C virus in HIV-positive and PrEP-using MSM in England. J Viral Hepat 2020; 27:721-730.

9. Roberts H, Jiles R, Harris AM et al. Incidence and Prevalence of Sexually Transmitted Hepatitis B, United States, 2013-2018. Sex Transm Dis 2021; 48:305-309.

10. Lockart I, Matthews GV, Danta M. Sexually transmitted hepatitis C infection; the evoluting epidemic in HIV-positive and HIV-negative MSM. Curr Op Infect Dis 2019;32 ;31-7 11. Husa P. Current view on hepatitis B diagnosis and therapy. Vnitr Lek 2021;67:48-50.

12. Busch K, Thime B. The natural history of chronic hepatitis B virus infections. Med Microbiol Immunol (Berl) 2015; 204: 5-10

13. Tu T, Douglas MW. Hepatitis B Virus Infection: From Diagnostics to Treatments.Viruses. 2020;12:1366. doi: 10.3390/v12121366.

14. Hyams KC. Risk of chronicity followign acute hepatitis B virus infections: a review. Clin infect Dis 1995; 20: 992-1000

15. He S, Lockart I, Alavi M et al. Systematic review with meta-analysis: effectiveness of direct-acting antiviral treatment for hepatitis C in patients with hepatocellular carcinoma. Aliment Pharmacol Ther 2020;51:34-52.

16. Westin J, Aleman S, Castedal M et al. Management of hepatitis B virus infection, updated Swedish guidelines. Infect Dis (Lond) 2020;52:1-22.

17. Baumert TF, Berg T, Lim JK et al. Status of direct-acting antiviral therapy for hepatitis C virus infection and remaining challenges. Gastroenterology 2019;156:431-445.

18. Nguyen MH, Wong G, Gane E et al. Hepatitis B Virus: Advances in Prevention, Diagnosis, and Therapy. Clin Microbiol Rev 2020;33:e00046-19. doi: 10.1128/CMR.00046-19

19. Rabaan AA, Al-Ahmed SH, Bazzi AM et al. Overview of hepatitis C infection, molecular biology, and new treatment.Infect Public Health. 2020;13:773-783.

20. Centers for Diseases Control and Prevention. Sexually transmitted infections treatement.

Guidelines 2021. MMR 2021; 70: 30-59

STIs and digestive disorders

In addition to infections by viral hepatitis viruses, which cause digestive problems, other intestinal agents that can be contracted during sexual intercourse have been described, particularly in certain exposed populations [1].

The transmission of Entamoeba histolytica, Enteromona hominis, Giadia, Lamblia, Shigella sonnei and S. flexneri, *Campylobacter jejuni* during sexual contact (ano-buccal or feco-oral) was documented in the 1970s, particularly in the population of men who have sex with men [2-4]. In fact, data shows that in this population group, the incidence of infection is 6 to 14% higher than in the general population or a control group. This shows the high risk of exposure to this type of infection [3]. Clinical manifestations are essentially dominated by intestinal signs (diarrhoea, abdominal colic) with no major complications apart from severe cases of dehydration due to acute diarrhoea [3, 4].

Treatment must be adapted to each type of microorganism. Increased resistance to several antibiotics has been described for Shigellosis infections, particularly in the USA (azithromycin ciprofloxacin) [5-7].

References

1. Newman KL, Newman GS, Cybulski RJ et al. Gastroenteritis in men who have sex with men in Seatle, Washington 2017,2018. Clin Infect Dis 2029; 71:109-115.

2. Wu HH, Shen YT, Chiuo CS et al. Shigellosis outbreak among MSM living with HIV: a case-control study in Taiwan, 2015-2016. Sex Transm Infect 2019; 95 :76-70

3. Richardson D, Devlin J, Fitzpatrick C et al. Sexually transmitted *Shigella flexneri* and *Shigella sonnei* in men who have sex with men. Sex Transm Infect 2021; 97:244. doi: 10.1136/sextrans-2020-054589.

4. Hung CC. Chang SY, Ji DD. Entamoeba hystolytica infection who sex with men. Lancet Infect Dis 2012; 12 : 729-36

5. Baker KS, Dalman TJ, Ashton PM et al. Intercontinental dissemination of azithromincin-resistant shigellosis through sexual transmission: a cross-sectional study. Lancet Infect Dis 2015 ;15 :193-21

6. Charles H, Prochazka M, Thorley K et al. Outbreak of sexually transmitted, extensively drugresistant Shigella sonnei in the UK, 2021-22: a descriptive epidemiological study. Lancet Infect Dis 2022; 22:1503-1510

7. Dallman TJ, Charles H, Prochazka M, et al. Emergence of novel strains of *Shigella flexneri* associated with sexual transmission in adult men in England, 2019-2020.
C.J Med Microbiol. 2021 Oct;70(10):001437. doi: 10.1099/jmm.0.001437.

Human scabiosis

1. Causal agent

Scabies is a highly contagious parasitic disease caused by *Sarcoptes scabiei hominis.* It has been shown that scabies appears mainly when there is a frequent change of partners [1].

Contamination occurs through direct contact, but also through contact with linen and bedding "it is mainly contracted in bed" [2]. Scabiosis is as common in men as in women. But it should be noted that scabies, which is extremely common in poor populations, is not primarily an STI, and is one of the neglected tropical diseases [3].

2. Symptomatology

The incubation period varies: usually 2 to 5 days, sometimes 1 to 2 weeks. The onset is marked by pruritus, mainly nocturnal [4-6]. This pruritus occurs in the interdigital spaces and on the sides of the fingers, the front of the armpits, the external genitals, the buttocks, and the extensor surfaces of the elbows and knees [5,6]. Within a few days, pruritus becomes generalised and increases in intensity. Examination reveals papulovesicular lesions, sometimes crusted, in the pruritic areas, with extensive scratching lesions. In the typical form, the characteristic scabious furrow may be found, appearing as a small, fine, sinuous, greyish line.

Pruritus and scratching lesions can lead to infectious complications (impetiginisation) [7]. Superinfected nodular and erosive lesions of the external genitalia are sometimes seen. Scabies in debilitated areas (elderly subjects, malignant haemopathy, therapeutic immunodepression, AIDS) may take on an erythematous-squamous, keratotic and nodular appearance (Norwegian scabies) [8-10]. Some authors have reported glomerular nephritis, which is often a complication secondary to streptococcal superinfection rather than a true complication of scabies.

3. Diagnosis

The nature of the pruritus, the possibility of infection and the appearance of the lesions are sufficient to make a diagnosis of scabies, especially during epidemic periods. The definitive diagnosis is based on the isolation of *Sarcoptes scabiei hominis* from the scales or furrows, using a microscope or dermoscopy [1, 2, 11, 12]. For public health purposes, diagnostic criteria have been established by the International Alliance for the Control of Scabies [13]. These criteria have been validated at the operational level by field health workers [14].

Table 13: International Alliance for the Control of Scabies diagnostic criteria [13].

A. Scabies confirmed	At least one of the following criteria present A2 larvae, eggs or faeces microscopically present on skin samples A2 mites, eggs or faeces visualised on an individual using a high-power imaging device A3, mites, eggs or faeces viewed on an individual using a dermatoscope
B. Clinical scabies	At least one of the following criteria is present B1 Scabious furrows B2 Typical lesions of the external genitalia in men B3 Typical lesions in typical locations and two historical forms
C. Suspected scabies	Presence of one of the following criteria Cl: Typical lesions in typical locations and a historical form C2: Atypical lesions or atypical locations and two historical forms
Historical forms	Hl: Pruritus H2: presence of any notion of contagion
The diagnosis is based on one of three criteria (A, B or C)	

Certain pruritic conditions may simulate scabiosis, as pruritus poses the problem of its multiple etiologies, in particular prurigo, larva migrans and pediculosis [1]. In the event of bacterial superinfection, primary impetigo, impetiginisation or impetiginised eczema should be discussed. Genital erosions may suggest chancre mou, herpes or syphilitic chancre [15]. These erosions may also be a gateway to other STDs, notably HIV infection.

4. Treatment

It must meet a dual objective: destroy the parasite and heal the skin lesions. The fundamental principle is to treat all the members of the same family or all the people in contact with them at the same time, on the same day. Curative treatment therefore involves disinfecting the body, linen and bedding.

- Disinfection of the body: local brushing of the whole body except the face with a solution of benzyl benzoate or permethrin in the evening at bedtime (to be kept on for 12 hours) for 2 to 3 consecutive evenings. There are no consensual recommendations as to the optimal regimen to adopt: one application or three applications? Repeat application after 8 days [16-19]. A recent study showed the efficacy of treatment with benzyl benzoate: one application per day repeated 08 days later with good clinical and parasitological clearance by day 28^{e} [20].
- Disinfection of linen and bedding: this is compulsory, and is carried out using powdered products - Oral ivermectin gives excellent results and is the drug of choice in mass treatment strategies [21-23], but the oral dose must be supplemented by disinfection of the bedding and linen

for greater effectiveness.

- Antibiotic therapy may be recommended in cases of severe impetiginisation.

References

1. Tarbox M, Walker K, Tan M. Scabies. JAMA 2018;320:612.
2. Thomas C, Coates SJ, Engelman D et al. Ectoparasites: Scabies. J Am Acad Dermatol. 2020; 82:533-548.
3. Leung AKC, Lam JM, Leong KF. Scabies: A Neglected Global Disease. Curr Pediatr Rev. 2020;16:33-42.
4. Chandler DJ, Fuller LC A Review of Scabies: An infestation more than skin deep. Dermatology 2019;235:79-90
5. Richards RN. Scabies: Diagnostic and therapeutic update. J Cutan Med Surg 2021;25:95- 101
6. Chosidow O. Clinical practices. Scabies. N Engl J Med 2006;354:1718-27.
7. Hay RJ, Steer AC, Engelman D et al. Scabies in the developing world: its prevalence, complications, and management.Clin Microbiol Infect. 2012;18:313-23
8. Pitche P, Wolkenstein P, Cremer G et al. Profuse scabies: kinetic curves of parasitologic cure with an association of benzyl benzoate and sulfiram. Ann Dermatol Venereol2002 ;129:287-9.
9. Govindarajan RK, Mitra S, Obiechina N et al. Norwegian scabies.Br J Hosp Med (Lond) 2013;74:471. doi: 10.12968/hmed.2013.74.8.471.
10. Pakanati K, Jagota D, Ladogana M. Norwegian scabies in HIV/AIDS. Proc (Bayl Univ Med Cent) 2022; 35:346-347
11. Micali G, Lacarrubba F, Verzi AE et al. Scabies: Advances in noninvasive diagnosis. PLoS Negl Trop Dis 2016;10:e0004691. doi: 10.1371/journal.pntd.0004691.
12. Thompson MJ, Engelman D, Gholam K et al. Systematic review of the diagnosis of scabies in therapeutic trials. Clin Exp Dermatol 2017;42:481-487
13. Engelman D, Yoshizumi J, Hay RJ et al. The 2020 International Alliance for the Control of Scabies Consensus Criteria for the Diagnosis of Scabies. Br J Dermatol 2020;183:808-820.
14. Walker SL, Collinson S, Timothy J et al. A community-based validation of the International Alliance for the Control of Scabies Consensus Criteria by expert and non-expert examiners in Liberia PLoS Negl Trop Dis.2020 ;14:e0008717. doi: 0.1371/journal.pntd.0008717.
15. Pitche P. Sexually transmitted ulcerations. EMC-Dermatologie 2022; 24 : 1-5 [article 98-450-A-10].
16. Thomas C, Rehmus W, Chang AY. Treatment practices in the management of scabies in infants younger than two months. Pediatr Dermatol 2021;38:431-435
17. Walker GJ, Johnstone PW. Interventions for treating scabies.
Cochrane Database Syst Rev 2000;(3):CD000320. doi: 10.1002/14651858.CD000320

17\. Lake SJ, Kaldor JM, Hardy M et al. Mass drug administration for the control of scabies: A systematic review and meta-analysis. Clin Infect Dis 2022;75:959-967.

18\. Widaty S, Miranda E, Cornain EF et al. Scabies: update on treatment and efforts for prevention and control in highly endemic settings. J Infect Dev Ctries 2022 ;16:244-251

19\. Bernigaud C, Fischer K, Chosidow O. The Management of Scabies in the 21st Century: past, advances and potentials. Acta Derm Venereol 2020;100:adv00112. doi: 10.2340/00015555-3468.

20\. Caumes E, Marty M, Cadot M et al. A prospective cohort of patients with common scabies treated with 10% benzyl benzoate emulsion as monotherapy: EPIGALE study.
Int J Dermatol 2022; 61:434-441.

21\. Ly F, Caumes E, Ndaw CA et al. Ivermectin versus benzyl benzoate applied once or twice to treat human scabies in Dakar, Senegal: a randomized controlled trial.
Bull World Health Organ 2009;87:424-30

22\. Meyersburg D, Welponer T, Kaiser A et al. Comparison of topical benzyl benzoate vs. oral ivermectin in treating scabies: A randomized study. J Eur Acad Dermatol Venereol 2023;37:160-165.

23. Hardy M, Samuela J, Kama M et al. Community control strategies for scabies: A cluster randomised noninferiority trial. PLoS Med 2021;18:e1003849. doi: 10.1371/journal.pmed.1003849. eCollection 2021

Pubic phthisis

1. Causal agent

Pubic lice is an infection caused by an insect of the order Anoplura [1]. Transmission occurs during sexual contact. The female lays eggs 24 hours after mating, and 3 eggs per day up to a maximum of 26 [1,2]. The larva matures between 13 and 17 days [1]. The adult insect has an average lifespan of 3 to 4 weeks [1].

2. Symptomatology

Pruritus remains the main symptom and is the reason for consultation. The pruritus is usually constant, but mostly recurs at night [3-5]. Pruritus is accompanied by scratching lesions. On examination, blood spots can be seen under the clothing, reflecting the crushing of blood-feeding insects. The preferred site is the pubis in both sexes. But blood spots can also be seen on other parts of the body (especially hairy areas), such as the thorax, thighs, axillae and scalp. In fact, when the hair grows, the nits remain attached [4, 5]. The main complication is bacterial superinfection of the scratch marks.

3. Diagnosis

The diagnosis is essentially clinical, as the eggs of adult insects can be seen. However, microscopic examination of the hair can confirm the diagnosis with certainty [1-3].

4. Treatment

It involves treating the patient and contacts with pediculicides [6-9]. The usual local medications are permethrin 1%, malathion 0.5%, benzyl benzoate 25% or ivermectin lotion 0.5%. Treatment with oral ivermectin is recommended in certain chronic or severe forms at a dosage of 200 to 400 ug/kg per day [8].

To prevent recurrence, bedding, clothing and underwear must be disinfected in all cases of contact (and even in those around them).

References

1. Ko CJ, Elston DM. Pediculosis. J Am Acad Dermatol 2004;50:1-12
2. Creighton-Smith M, Sloan SB. Pediculosis Pubis. JAMA Dermatol 2019;155:1416
3. Chuard C. Pediculosis. Rev Med Suisse 2007;3:2266
4. Chosidow O. Scabies and pediculosis. Lancet 2000;355:819-26
5. Coates SJ, Thomas C, Chosidow O et al. Ectoparasites: Pediculosis and tungiasis. J Am Acad Dermatol 2020;82:551-56
6. Gunning K, Pippitt K, Kiraly B et al. Pediculosis and scabies: treatment update. Am Fam Physician 2012;86 :535-41.
7. Mumcuoglu KY, Pollack RJ, Reed DL et al. International recommendations for an effective control of head louse infestations. Int J Dermatol 2021;60:272-280.
8. Salavastru CM, Chosidow O, Janier M et al. GS. European guideline for the management of pediculosis pubis J Eur Acad Dermatol Venereol 2017;31:1425-1428
9. Leone PA. Scabies and pediculosis pubis: an update of treatment regimens and general review. Clin Infect Dis 2007;44 (Suppl 3):S153-9

Molluscum contagiosum

1. Causal agent

Molluscum contagiosum (MC) is a viral infection caused by a poxvirus in the same family as smallpox, and two strains are known (MCV 1 and MCV2) [1, 2]. It is a benign infection and relatively common in children. Molluscum contagiosum is mainly contracted through direct or indirect contact with bedding or clothing [1]. The identification of MC as a sexually transmitted disease dates back to the 1970s. In the 80s and 90s, an increase in the number of cases of CD associated with HIV infection was observed in both children and adults. In fact, the factors that favour or increase the susceptibility of adults to this infection are HIV-related immunodepression and malnutrition [3-4]. In patients infected with HIV-1, the prevalence of clinical MCV infection is 5-18% [3]. In young adults, sexual intercourse is the most likely form of transmission and genital lesions are the most common. Oral and peribuccal lesions resulting from sexual transmission are also possible, especially in immunocompromised patients.

2. Symptomatology

After an incubation period of between 2 weeks and 3 months, hemispherical translucent papules of variable size and umbilication appear. This cupuliform umbilication is quite evocative clinically. In 1ST, the first lesions appear in the genital area (pubis and external genitalia), but can also be seen on the thighs and trunk [4-7]. In immunocompromised (HIV) patients, there are profuse forms on the trunk and face [7].

3. Diagnosis

Positive diagnosis is easily made clinically, based on the history of the disease and the umbilical features of the lesions. The diagnosis is clinical, but can be confirmed by histopathological or cytogenetic examinations or by PCR (DNA viruses). Dermatoscopy has recently been proposed as a non-invasive technique for diagnosing atypical forms of CD, particularly in adults [1, 2]. In practice, the differential diagnosis is made with warts, monkeypox lesions, acne, lichen planus and lichen striatus, depending on the location [1].

4. Treatment

Depending on the number of lesions, there are several therapeutic methods available in practice: curettage, which involves cutting the lesion very precisely with a curette; cryotherapy using liquid nitrogen; treatment with laser, immunoquimod 1% or salicylic acid [5, 8, 9]. In the case of HIV-related immunodepression, antiretrovirals restore the immune system, helping to achieve healing and prevent recurrence [8].

References.

1. Chen X, Anstey AV, Bugert JJ. Molluscum contagiosum virus infection. Lancet Infect Dis 2013;13:877-88.

2. Hanson D, Dayna G Diven G. Molluscum contagiosum. Dermatol Online J 2003;9:2-6

3. Rugpao S, Wanapirak C, Sirichotiyakul S et al. Sexually transmitted disease prevalence in brothel-based commercial sex workers in Chiang Mai, Thailand: impact of the condom use campaign. J Med Assoc Thai 1997;80:426-30.

4. Chopra A, Mittal RR, Singh P et al. Pattern of sexually transmitted diseases at Patiala. Indian J Sex Transm Dis 1990;11:43-5.

5. Martin P. Interventions for molluscum contagiosum in people infected with human immunodeficiency virus: a systematic review. Int J Dermatol 2016;55:956-66.

6. Silverman RF, Shinder R. Molluscum Contagiosum. N Engl J Med 2022;386:582.

7. Gur I. The epidemiology of Molluscum contagiosum in HIV-seropositive patients: a unique entity or insignificant finding? Int J STD AIDS 2008;19:503-6

8. van der Wouden JC, van der Sande R, Kruithof EJ et al. Interventions for cutaneous molluscum contagiosum. Cochrane Database Syst Rev 2017;5:CD004767. doi: 10.1002/14651858.CD004767

9. Badavanis G, Pasmatzi E, Monastirli A et al. Topical Imiquimod is an Effective and Safe Drug for Molluscum Contagiosum in Children. Acta Dermatovenerol Croat 2017; 25:164-166.

PART V

V. Re-emerging and emerging sexually transmitted infections

1ST reemergents

Over the last twenty years, Europe and the USA have seen the re-emergence of epidemics of certain germs (N. *meningitis)* and/or certain STIs (such as venereal lymphogranulomatosis), the prevalence of which had fallen sharply in the 1980s-1990s in northern countries [1, 2].

1. Neisseria meningitidis (NM) infection

Classically, this germ colonises the nasopharyngeal sphere and is responsible for epidemics of cerebrospinal meningitis in tropical countries, particularly in Africa. In the past, cases of NM urethritis have been described in heterosexuals and MSM [2,3].

Since 2015, there have been reports of an increasingly high incidence of NM urethritis among MSM in the USA [2], with small epidemics occurring in clusters in certain cities and STI screening clinics. Transmission is likely to occur through oral-sexual contact [3]. Cases of genuine meningitis associated with urethritis have been reported. Indeed, between 2012 and 2015, 74 cases of meningitis were reported in MSM whose mode of contamination was sexual [3-5]. In the USA, the NM serotype observed is group C. The vulnerability factors of these cases of sexual infection of NM with meningitis are not well documented: an associated factor such as HIV infection has been suggested [5]. Treatment for *N. meningitidis* urethritis is based on ceftriaxone, as for NG urethritis.

2. Lymphogranulomatosis venereum

LGV is caused by the L1 L2 L3 serovars of Chlamydia trachomatis. Although the infection is endemic in tropical countries, its prevalence fell sharply in northern countries in the 1990s. In northern countries, a resurgence of LGV was noted in the early 2000s [6]. Since 2003, Europe and the United States have reported high incidences of clustered LGV in MSM groups. Between 2014 and 2016, more than 10,000 cases of LGV were reported in Europe [6, 7]. The clinical manifestations of LGV are dominated by rectal syndrome [7, 8]. The associated risk factors are receptive anal intercourse and associated HIV infection. Treatment is the same as for classical LGV, with cyclins as the first-line treatment.

3. Mycoplasma genitalium (MG) infections

MG has long been considered a commensal germ of the genital mucosa. It was first considered to be an STI germ when it was isolated from a man suffering from non-gonococcal urethritis [9]. In recent years, with the routine use of molecular biology (PCR) in the diagnosis and screening of genital discharges, MG has increasingly been isolated as the cause of non-gonococcal urethritis and certain cervicitis [10]. However, it is not recommended to actively screen for these conditions. A major problem with this infection is the increasing emergence of strains of MG that are resistant to macrolides, particularly azithromycin [11, 12].

References

1. Williamson D, Chen MY. Emerging and reemergieng sexually transmistted infections. NEJM 2020;182 :2023-32
2. Janda WN, Bohnoff M, Morello JA et al. Prevalence and site-pathogen studies of Nesseiria meninigitidis and Nesseiria gonorhoeoae in homosexual men. JAMA 1980; 244:2060-4
3. Bazan JA, Turner AN, Kircaldy RD et al. Large cluster of Neisseria meningitidis urethritis in Columbus, Ohio 2015, Clin Infect Dis 2017;65 :92-9
4. Kamiya H, MacNell J, Blain A et al. Meningococcocal disease among men who have sex with men. United States. January 2012-June 2015. MMWR 2015 ; 64 :1256-7
5. Ma KC, Unemo M, Jeveira S et al. Genomic characterization of urethritis-associated Neisseria meningitidis show that a wide range of N. menigitidis strains can cause urethritis. J Clin

Microbiol 2017; 55:3374-83
6. Prochazka M, Charles H, Allen H et al. Rapid increase in lymphogranuloma venereum among HIV-Negative men who have sex with men, England, 2019.
Emerg Infect Dis. 2021;27:2695-2699.
7. Bissessor M Fairley CK Timothy Read T et al.The etiology of infectious proctitis in men who have sex with men differs according to HIV status. Sex Transm Dis 2013; 40:768-70.
8. De Vries HJC. Lymphogranuloma venereum in werstern world, 15 years after its reemergernce;
new perspectives and reaserch priorities? Curr Opin Infect Dis 2019;32:49-50
9. Tully JG, Taylor-Robinson D, Cole RM et al. A newly discorvered mycoplasma in the Mycoplasma human urogenital tract. Lancet 1981;1:1288-91
10. Gnanadurai R, Fifer H. *Mycoplasma genitalium:* A Review. Microbiology (Reading) 2020;166:21-29.
11. Martens L, Kuster S, de Vos et al. Macrolide-Resistant Mycoplasma genitalium in Southeastern Region of Netherland, 2014-2017. Emerg Infect Dis 2019;25:1297-1303
12. Hokynar K, Hiltunen-Back E, Mannonen L et al. Prevalence of *Mycoplasma genitalium* and mutations associated with macrolide and fluoroquinolone resistance in Finland. *Int J STD AIDS 2018 ; 29 :904-907.*

1ST emergent

1. The Zika Virus

Pathogen

Zika fever is caused by an arbovirus belonging to the *Flaviviridae* family, *of the flavivirus* genus, like the dengue and yellow fever viruses [1]. The insect that carries the disease is the female mosquito of the genus *Aedes*, which can be identified by the black and white stripes on its legs [1]. The species currently capable of transmitting the Zika virus is *Aedes aegypti, which* originates from Africa [2]. *The Aedes albopictus* (tiger mosquito, native to Asia) could also prove to be a vector of the Zika virus, as it already is for dengue fever and chikungunya [3]. The mosquito is infected with the virus during a blood meal, when it bites a person carrying Zika. The virus multiplies within the mosquito without consequence for the insect. Then, the next time it bites, the mosquito releases the virus into the bloodstream of a new person. Symptoms appear 3 to 12 days after the bite, but during this time the person may infect other mosquitoes if bitten again [2].
In recent epidemics, cases of sexual transmission of the Zika virus have been reported [4, 5]. The virus has been found in saliva, sperm and vaginal secretions. The median time for elimination of the virus in semen is 42 days, with 95% elimination at 4 months [5]. However, it should be stressed that in epidemic areas, it is difficult to estimate the risk of purely sexual transmission from transmission by mosquitoes. The risk of sexual transmission is easier to assess in non-epidemic areas, in couples where one of the partners has just returned from a trip to an endemic area. To reduce this risk, the World Health Organisation (WHO) has made the following recommendation: men and women should use condoms 3 and 2 months respectively after exposure to the Zika virus [6]. A pregnant woman and her sexual partner must use a condom throughout the pregnancy, because if the woman is infected, there is a risk of infection of the fetus and the newborn (the newborn's infection is the most serious aspect of this infection, with a risk of fetopathy).

Symptomatology

It is an influenza-like syndrome with headache, fever, arthralgias, myalgias and cough. This syndrome is associated with skin signs such as maculopapular exanthema [2]. A typical Guillan-Barre picture has been described [2]. In children infected during pregnancy, microcephaly is observed.

Diagnosis

It is based on epidemiological (epidemic, return from epidemic zone), clinical and above all paraclinical arguments. This involves identifying the Zika virus (RNA virus) using molecular biology (PCR) [1, 3].

Treatment

Zika virus disease is generally relatively benign and requires no specific treatment. People who are infected and symptomatic should rest, drink enough fluids and take medication for pain and fever [2]. If symptoms worsen, they should consult an appropriate care centre. There is currently no vaccine available.

Prevention

Protection against mosquito bites is an essential measure for preventing Zika virus infection [2]. This can be achieved by applying repellent products, wearing clothing (preferably light-coloured) that covers as much of the body as possible, installing physical barriers such as insect screens, closing doors and windows, sleeping under mosquito nets, and using repellent products [2, 6]. Particular attention should be paid to those who may not be able to protect themselves effectively, such as young children, the sick or the elderly. Pregnant women living in high-risk areas should protect themselves from mosquito bites by all these means, especially during the first two trimesters of pregnancy when the risk of fatal malformations is greatest [2, 6]. It is also important to empty or clean all potential mosquito breeding sites, such as buckets, cans, flower pots, gutters and used tyres.

2. Ebola virus

Pathogen

The Ebola virus disease first appeared in 1976, during 2 simultaneous outbreaks in Nzara (now in South Sudan) and Yambuku (Democratic Republic of Congo) [7]. Yambuku is located near the Ebola River, which gave its name to the disease. The disease occurs endemo-epidemically in Equatorial Africa, with the Democratic Republic of Congo remaining the epicentre [8]. The 2014-2016 outbreak in West Africa was the largest and most complex since the virus was discovered in 1976 [9-12]. It produced more cases and deaths than all previous outbreaks combined.

The Filoviridae family of viruses comprises 3 genera: Cuevavirus, Marburgvirus and Ebolavirus. Five species have been identified in Ebolavirus: Zaire, Bundibugyo, Sudan, Reston and Foret de Tai' [13]. The first 3 have been associated with major outbreaks in Africa. The virus responsible for the 2014-2016 outbreak in West Africa belongs to the Zaire species [10]. Fruit bats of the Pteropodidae family are thought to be the natural hosts of the Ebola virus. The virus enters the human population after close contact with the blood, secretions, organs or biological fluids of infected animals such as chimpanzees, gorillas, fruit bats, monkeys, wood antelopes or porcupines found sick or dead in tropical forests.

During the epidemic in West Africa between 2014 and 2016, the Ebola virus was identified in the semen of survivors [14-19]. In a prospective study, the median survival of viral RNA was 158 days [17]. The existence of sexual transmission of the virus led the WHO to propose that a PCR test be carried out in men's semen three months after recovery [19]. During this period, and as long as the test is positive, he should systematically use condoms during sexual intercourse.

Symptomatology

The first symptoms are febrile fatigue with a sudden onset, muscle pain, headache and sore throat [7, 11, 12]. These are followed by vomiting, diarrhoea, skin rash, symptoms of renal and hepatic failure and, in some cases, internal and external bleeding (e.g. bleeding gums, blood in stools) [11, 12].

Diagnosis

Diagnosis is made using molecular biology. Automated or semi-automated nucleic acid tests (NATs) are available for routine diagnostic management [11, 12].

Treatment

Supportive oral or intravenous rehydration and symptomatic treatment tailored to the individual patient improve survival rates [7, 12]. No specific curable treatment is currently available for

Ebola virus disease. However, a range of potential treatments, including blood products, immune therapies and drug treatments, are currently being evaluated. There is an effective Ebola vaccine (Ervebo) that protects against this deadly virus as part of the fight against this infection [20, 21].

3. Monkey pox

Monkeypox (or simian orthopoxvirosis) is a viral zoonosis (virus transmitted to humans by animals) whose symptoms are less severe than those observed in smallpox patients in the past [22].

Pathogen

The monkeypox virus is a double-stranded DNA envelope virus belonging to the Orthopoxvirus genus of the Poxviridae family [22]. There are two distinct genetic clades of monkeypox virus: the Central African clade (Congo Basin) and the West African clade [22, 24, 26]. Several animal species are susceptible to monkeypox virus. These include funisciurs, squirrels, savannah cricetomes, dormice, primates and other species [27]. Transmission from animals to humans (zoonotic) can result from direct contact with blood, biological fluids or skin or mucous lesions from infected animals. In Africa, there is evidence of monkeypox virus infection in many animals, including funisciurs, squirrels, savannah cricetomes and some monkey species [22, 23].

Consumption of meat and other products from infected animals without sufficient cooking is a possible risk factor [24]. Human-to-human transmission may result from close contact with secretions from the respiratory tract or skin lesions of an infected individual, or with objects that have been recently contaminated [23]. Transmission can also occur through close contact during and after childbirth.

Although close physical contact is a well-known risk factor for transmission, it is not yet clear that monkeypox can be transmitted specifically via genital secretions, even though the last epidemics in Europe in 2021 and 2022 occurred in the population of men who have sex with men [27-31]. Cases contracted during heterosexual intercourse have also been reported [32].

Symptomatology

The incubation period (the interval between infection and the appearance of symptoms) generally varies from 6 to 13 days, but may be as short as 5 to 21 days. Infection can be divided into two periods [31]. The invasive period (lasting from 0 to 5 days) is characterised by the appearance of fever, intense headache, adenopathy, back pain, myalgia and marked asthenia [29]. The rash usually begins within 1-3 days of the onset of fever. It is generally more concentrated on the face and extremities than on the trunk [31]. It affects the face (in 95% of cases) and the palms of the hands and soles of the feet (in 75% of cases). The oral mucosa (in 70% of cases), genitals (30%) and conjunctivae (20%), as well as the horn, are also affected [31, 32]. The eruption progresses in the following order [31]: macules (lesions with a flattened base), papules (firm lesions in slight relief), vesicles (lesions filled with clear fluid), pustules (lesions filled with yellowish fluid) and finally crusts that dry out and fall off. The number of lesions can range from a few to several thousand. In severe cases, the lesions may coalesce until large flaps of skin detach [33].

Monkeypox usually resolves spontaneously, with symptoms lasting from 2 to 4 weeks [29]. Severe cases occur more frequently in children and are related to the extent of exposure to the virus, the patient's state of health and the nature of the complications [29, 31]. Underlying immunodeficiency can lead to an unfavourable course. Complications of monkeypox include secondary infections, bronchopneumonia, septicaemia, encephalitis and infection of the cornea, which may lead to loss of vision [29]. The incidence of monkeypox has traditionally ranged from 0 to 11% in the general population, with higher rates in young children [33].

Diagnosis

Molecular biology tests allow rapid diagnosis. The polymerase chain reaction (PCR) is the preferred laboratory test because of its accuracy and sensitivity [33, 34]. The optimal diagnostic samples for monkeypox are those taken from skin lesions, tissues or fluid from vesicles and pustules, and dry crusts. PCR analysis of blood samples is generally negative due to the short duration of the viremia, which depends on the time at which samples are collected after the onset of symptoms, and it is not recommended to collect them systematically from patients [33]. The differential diagnosis should take into account other eruptive diseases, such as chickenpox, measles, bacterial skin infections, scabies, syphilis and drug allergies [35-37].

Treatment

Clinical care is purely asymptotic (disinfection of lesions, antibiotic therapy in the event of superinfection). Secondary bacterial infections should be treated with antibiotics tailored to the sites of infection [29, 38]. An antiviral agent known as tecovirimat is thought to be effective against infection [39-41]. If used to treat patients, tecovirimat should ideally be monitored in a clinical research setting with prospective data collection.

Vaccination

Vaccination against the disease is an effective means of preventing transmission [42, 43]. Some countries offer a vaccine to people likely to be at risk: men who have sex with men, sex workers, laboratory staff, rapid response teams and health workers.

References

1. Chong HY, Leow CY, Abdul Majeed AB et al. Flavivirus infection-A review of immunopathogenesis, immunological response, and immunodiagnosis.Virus Res 2019;274:197770. doi: 10.1016/j.virusres.2019.197770. Epub 2019 Oct 15
2. Baud D, Gubler DJ, Schaub B et al. An update on Zika virus infection. Lancet 201;390:2099-2109.
3. Castro-Amarante MF, Pereira SS, Pereira LR et al. The anti-dengue virus peptide DV2 inhibits Zika Virus both in vitro and in vivo. Viruses 2023;15:839. doi: 10.3390/v15040839.
4. Musso D, Roche C, Robin E et al. Potential sexual transmission of Zika virus. N Engl J Med 2016 ;374 :2195-8
5. Moreira J, Peisoto TM, Siquiera AM et al. Sexually acquired Zika virus: a systematic review. Clin Microbiol Infect 2017 ;23 :296-305
6. World Health Organisation. Guidelines for the prevention of sexual transmission of Zika virus. Geneva 2019
7. Nicastri E, Kobinger G, Vairo F et al. Ebola Virus Disease: Epidemiology, clinical features, management, and prevention. Infect Dis Clin North Am 2019;33:953-976.
8. Green A. DR Congo: investigational research against Ebola virus. Lancet 2018;391:2308-2309.
9. Arwady MA, Bawo L, Hunter JC et al. Evolution of ebola virus disease from exotic infection to global health priority, Liberia, mid-2014. Emerg Infect Dis2015;21:578-84
10. Holmes EC, Dudas G, Rambaut A et al The evolution of Ebola virus: Insights from the 2013-2016 epidemic. Nature 2016;538:193-200
11. Malvy D, McElroy AK, de Clerck H et al Ebola virus disease. Lancet. 2019;393:936-948.
12. Feldmann H, Sprecher A, Geisbert TW. Ebola. N Engl J Med 2020;382:1832-1842.
13. Dolzhikova IV, Shcherbinin DN, Logunov DY et al. Ebola virus *(Filoviridae: Ebolavirus: Zaire ebolavirus'):* fatal adaptation mutations. Vopr Virusol 2021;66:7-16.
14. Sissoko D, Duraffour S, Kerber R et al. Persistence and clearence of Ebola virus RNA from seminal fluid of Ebola virus disease survivors: a longitidinal analysis and modeling study. Lancet Glob Health 2017 ;5 :e80-88
15. Vetter P, Fischer WA 2nd, Schibler M et al. Ebola virus shedding and transmission: review of current evidence. J Infect Dis 2016;214(suppl 3):S177-S184
16. Thorson A, Formenty P, Lofthouse C et al. Systematic review of the literature on viral persistence and sexual transmission from recovered Ebola survivors: evidence and recommendations. BMJ Open 2016;6:e008859. doi: 10.1136/bmjopen-2015-008859.
17. Abbate JL, Murall CL, Richner H et al. Potential impact of sexual transmission on Ebola Virus epidemiology: Sierra Leone as a Case Study. PLoS Negl Trop Dis 2016;10:e0004676. doi: 10.1371/journal.pntd.0004676. eCollection 2016

18. Den Boon S, Marston BJ, Nyenswah TG et al. Ebola virus infection associated with transmission from survivors. Emerg Infect Dis 2019;25:249-255
19. Mate SE, Kugleman JR, Nyenwsh TG et al. Molecular evidence of sexual transmission of Ebola virus. N Engl J Med 2015 ;373 :2448-54
20. Tomori O, Kolawole MO. Ebola virus disease: current vaccine solutions. Curr Opin Immunol. 2021;71:27-33
21. Medaglini D, Santoro F, Siegrist CA. Correlates of vaccine-induced protective immunity against Ebola virus disease. Semin Immunol. 2018;39:65-72.
22. Di Giulio DB, Eckburg PB. Human monkeypox: an emerging zoonosis. Lancet Infect Dis. 2004;4:15-25
23. Karagoz A, Tombuloglu H, Alsaeed M et al. Monkeypox (mpox) virus: Classification, origin, transmission, genome organization, antiviral drugs, and molecular diagnosis. J Infect Public Health 2023;16:531-541
24. Mauldin MR, McCollum AM, Nakazawa YJ et al. Exportation of Monkeypox virus from the African continent. J Infect Dis 2022;225:1367-1376.
25. Rimoin AW, Kabela R, Ilunga B et al. Endemic human monkeypox in Democratic Republic of Congo: 2001-2004. Emerg Infect Dis 2007 ;13 ;934-7
26. Alakunle E, Moens U, Nchinda G et al. Monkeypox virus in Nigeria: infection biology, epidemiology, and evolution. Viruses 2020;12:1257. doi: 10.3390/v12111257
27. Falendysz EA, Lopera JG, Rocke TE. Monkeypox virus in animals: current knowledge of viral transmission and pathogenesis in wild animal reservoirs and captive animal models. Viruses 2023;15:905. doi: 10.3390/v15040905.
28. Vusirikala A, Charles H, Balasegaram S et al. Epidemiology of early Monkeypox virus transmission in sexual networks of gay and bisexual men, England, 2022. Emerg Infect Dis 2022;28:2082-2086.
29. Gessain A. Nakoune E, Yazdanpanah Y et al. Monkeypox. N Engl J Med 2022; 10;387:1783-1793
30. Curran KG, Eberly K, Russel OO et al. HIV and sexually transmistted infections in persons with monkeypox MMWR 2022; 71 :1141-7
31. Petersen E, Kantele A, Koopmans M et al. Human monkeypox: epidemiologic and clinical characteristics, diagnosis, and prevention. Infect Dis Clin North Am 2019;33:1027-1043
32. Ogoina D, Irebewule JHn Ogunleye A et al. The 2017 human monkeypox experience and response in the Niger Delta University Teaching hospital. Bayelsa State, Nigeria. PlosOne 2019;14 :e0214229
33. Altindis M, Puca E, Shapo L. Diagnosis of monkeypox virus - An overview. Travel Med Infect Dis 2022; 50:102459.
34. Li Y, Zhao H, Wilkins K et al. Real-time PCR assays for the specific detection of monkeypox virus West African and Congo Basin strain DNA. J Virol Methods 2010;169:223- 7.
35. Catala A, Clavo-Escribano P, Riera-Monroig J et al. Monkeypox outbreak in Spain: clinical and epidemiological findings in a prospective cross-sectional study of 185 cases. Br J Dermatol 2022;187:765-772.
36. Gupta AK, Talukder M, Rosen T et al. Differential Diagnosis, Prevention, and Treatment of mpox (Monkeypox): A Review for Dermatologists Am J Clin Dermatol 2023: 27:1-16.
37. Frew JW. Monkeypox: Cutaneous clues to clinical diagnosis. J Am Acad Dermatol 2023;88:698-700
38. Rizk JG, Lippi G, Henry BM et al. Prevention and treatment of Monkeypox. Drugs 2022;82:957-963.
39. Sherwat A, Brooks JT, Birnkrant D et al. Tecovirimat and the treatment of monkeypox: past, present, and future considerations. N Engl J Med 2022;387:579-581.
40. Mbrenga F, Nakoune E, Malaka C et al. Tecovirimat for monkeypox in Central African

Republic under expanded access. N Engl J Med 2022;387:2294-2295.
41. Desai AN, Thompson GR 3rd, Neumeister SM et al. Compassionate use of Tecovirimat for the treatment of monkeypox infection. JAMA 2022;32:1348-1350
42. Petersen BW, Kabamba J, McCollum AM et al. Vaccinating against monkeypox in the Democratic Republic of the Congo. Antiviral Res 2019;162:171-177.
43. Deputy NP, Deckert J, Chard AN et al. Vaccine effectiveness of JYNNEOS against mpox disease in the United States. N Engl J Med 2023 ; doi: 10.1056/NEJMoa2215201

PART VI

VI. 1ST and mental leap

STIs and psychosomatic symptoms

1. Circumstances of onset

There are two circumstances in which this occurs:

- The symptoms appear after an episode of infection or lesions of the urethro-genital system. In fact, a trivial lesion can lead to reactive anxiety [1]. Psychosomatic symptoms may be secondary to treatment failure or frequent recurrence (herpes), or in the event of sequelae (urethral stenosis, indelible scarring from a soft chancre) [2].
- Psychosomatic manifestations may be primitive (with no antecedent or episode of STI). Manifestations of venereophobia appear after a lapse in sexual activity, during unprotected sex, or after reading, talking, watching a medical programme on the radio or television, or on social networks [3].

2. Symptomatology

Whatever the circumstances of onset, the clinical pictures differ from one individual to another. Men mainly consult for meatic or urethral burning, sometimes for abnormal wetness of the duct or for penile or testicular pain; cloudy urine can increase anxiety [4]. Women complain of pain on micturition or even permanent pain, vulvar burning or dyspareunia [4, 5]. Vaginal touching is sometimes impossible. In both sexes, these patients are often psychasthenic, localising their anxiety or remorse in the urethro-vaginal sphere. In men, the "painful perineo-spermatic syndrome", equivalent to the "cystalgia with clear urine" syndrome in women, has been described by certain authors [3].

Numerous clinical forms can be observed [6, 7]:

- form with hypomanic excitement, associated with sexual hyperactivity and accompanied by psycho-characteristic disorders;
- forms with depressive reactions ranging from anxious melancholia to depressive somatic equivalents. The fear of infecting their family and friends or becoming sterile often leads patients to take several antibiotics and change doctors frequently.

The frequency of these manifestations is difficult to assess, particularly in the general population and in patients who already have or have had an STI [5-8].

Special cases of psycho-sexual illnesses

According to Tordjman [9, 10], the history of societies shows that unlike other diseases, 1STs have been accompanied by two particular signs: shame and social stigmatisation. For some individuals, the repercussions of STIs go beyond the purely somatic sphere (complications) and include the perception of the disease and society's assumed view of risky sexual behaviour [9]. Indeed, most STIs, like all diseases affecting the genitals, have been invested with symbolic power since the dawn of time (with mythological, religious and social quotations) and are accompanied by a feeling of devaluation and self-depreciation [10]. Depressive reactions, whether overt or hidden behind psychosomatic manifestations (insomnia, anorexia, fatigue, genital pain), are all accompanied by a loss of interest in sexuality.

1ST often causes sexual dysfunction, with altered sexual interest or lack of desire [10]. In women, anorgasmia, especially coital anorgasmia, secondary vaginismus or dyspareunia, and functional or psychogenic pain during penetration are often noted; in men, painful ejaculation or premature ejaculation are sequelae of poorly treated prostatitis. In both sexes, recurrent herpes poisons individual sexuality and especially that of the couple [11, 12]. Condylomata acuminata affect self-esteem and body image, and often lead to sexual dysfunction [12].

Tordjman identifies several psychological personalities on the basis of the repercussions depending on the type of individual [10].

The culprit: the anxious and ashamed patient. In fact, the mere mention of the word STI (syphilis, HIV for example) is enough to arouse feelings of fear, and the patient is racked with worry and guilt ever since he noticed a suspicious sign in his genitals. This sometimes leads to decisions to abstain radically until they are cured.

It *terrorises* him. This is the person who develops an irrational fear of 1STs. They are very well informed through the media about all STIs and their treatments, and are on the lookout for any infra-clinical or biological signs that might alert them. They may develop a phobia of sexuality and an obsession with STIs.

The masochist. As soon as he engages in sexual behaviour that is deemed to be risky (sometimes wrongly), he undergoes multiple biological tests, the negative results of which (HIV serology or syphilis, for example) leave him speechless. He awaits the biological punishment as the just chastisement for his sin and the sign of his unworthiness.

The matcho, the narcissist and the blase. The macho man wears his STD as a sign of virility.

The narcissist appreciates the attention lavished on him by the medical team (he asks for consultations and can multiply them at will). The blase sees his condition as a risk inherent in his lifestyle (others are prepared not to change their risky behaviour because they willingly accept the consequences).

In addition to these individual profiles, the Munchhausen syndrome can be observed: these are patients who complain of feigned STIs and report urethral discharge, genital erosions and dyspareunia, both to attract the practitioner's attention and to fuel their marital conflicts. Of course, all the practical examinations are normal and patients may have multiple consultations with several specialists. Practitioners need to be aware of this kind of psychopathological context in order to refer patients for appropriate treatment.

Impact on the couple

The occurrence of an STI in a couple leads to feelings of doubt, anxiety and mistrust, particularly in their love life [9]. Certain recurrent STIs such as herpes, condylomata or mycosis are a slow poison and can lead to a break-up.

The problems of dyspareunia and loss of sexual desire are sources of frustration and conflict in the couple that the doctor must understand and explain and, if possible, propose appropriate treatment by specialists.

3. Diagnosis

The diagnosis of psychosomatic manifestations during STIs is one of elimination [3, 11]. In fact, all infectious etiologies must first be investigated, before a psychological investigation is instituted. The necessary tests should be carried out to rule out :

- microbial etiology (parasitic, mycological, bacterial or viral) ;
- a local congenital or acquired anomaly of the uretero-genital system (uretrorraphy and echotomography may sometimes be necessary);
- a neighbouring pathology.

The psychological interview should consist of listening carefully to the patient's story (take time, and let the patient tell his whole story, which should not be trivialised). This guided conversation should include details of the patient's family and professional life.

4. Treatment

- Psychotherapy. This is the basis of all treatment, and depends essentially on the conclusions of the psychological investigation [12]. It allows the patient to be given logical explanations, to regain confidence by explaining the particularities of his ureterogenital condition, and by making him understand that his guilt is not necessarily real. You should not hesitate to refer the patient to a real psychotherapist or psychiatrist, or to ensure that the patient is cared for in a multidisciplinary setting.
- Sedatives or mild anxiolytics are sometimes essential to help patients get through the difficult phase. However, it is important not to give in easily to the patient's request for a prescription [12]

and to know how to refer the patient for psychological or psychiatric follow-up, depending on the case.

References

1. Goens J. De la syphilis au Sida, cinq siecles de m emoires litteraires de Venus. Presses Universitaires europeennes. Brussels, 1995

2. Bajos N, Bozon M Giami A et al. La sexualite aux temps de Sida. PUF, Paris 1998.

3. Gates JK, Gomez J. Venereophobia. Br J Hosp Med1984;31:435-6.

5. Magidson JF, Blashill AJ, Wall MM et al. Relationship between psychiatric disorders and sexually transmitted diseases in a nationally representative sample. Psychosom Res 2014;76:322-

6. Daubert E, French AL, Burgess HJ et al. Association of poor sleep with depressive and anxiety symptoms by HIV disease status: women's interagency HIV study. J Acquir Immune Defic Syndr 2022;89:222-230.

7. Arkell J, Osborn DP, Ivens D et al. Factors associated with anxiety in patients attending a sexually transmitted infection clinic: qualitative survey. Int J STD AIDS 2006;17:299-303

8. Osborn DP, King MB, Weir M. Psychiatric health in a sexually transmitted infections clinic: effect on reattendance. J Psychosom Res 2002;52 :267-72.

9. Tordjman G. La sexualite au fil de la vie. Hachette pratique, Paris 1996.

10. Tordjman G. In: Maux secrets. MST, Maladies taboues. Editions Autrement 1999, Paris

11. Morrison MF, Petitto JM, Ten Have T et al. Depressive and anxiety disorders in women with HIV infection. Am J Psychiatry 2002;159:789-96.

12. Paille M. La peau, le sexe et les mots : MST et Somatisation. In Maux secrets. MST, maladies taboues. Editions Autrement 1999, Paris

Psychiatric manifestations in HIV-infected patients

Mental illness increases the vulnerability of HIV-infected people and at the same time constitutes a risk factor for the acquisition of STIs [1-4]. It should also be emphasised that HIV infection and syphilis can, independently of each other, lead to psychiatric illness during the course of the disease, through damage to the central nervous system [5, 6].

1. STI/HIV-induced psychiatric disorders

Neurosyphilis may manifest as a psychiatric syndrome with irritability, mood disorders including depression and dementia [5, 7]. In practice, the clinical context and the history of the patient and the disease help to guide the etiological diagnosis, which will be confirmed by serological tests.

HIV infection can lead to psychiatric disorders in 10-60% of cases, depending on the study and the population subgroup [8-13]. The prevalence of psychiatric manifestations is higher in PLHIV than in the general population [14]. They take the form of cognitive impairment, depression and dementia [15-17]. These psychiatric manifestations are secondary to the chronic inflammation of the nervous system caused by HIV infection [11]. In addition, during the course of HIV infection, there are reports of genuine progressive multifocal leukoencephalopathy (PML) and cerebrovascular accidents (the sequelae of which may lead to vascular dementia) [9, 16]. The frequency of manifestations is higher in people aged over 50, and these manifestations are associated with the degree of immunodepression [16]. In fact, several studies have shown a significant drop in the prevalence of psychiatric symptoms in people living with HIV who are effectively treated with antiretroviral drugs, documenting the independent action of this infection in the development of these types of symptoms [3, 12, 28].

2. Psychiatric manifestations in PLHIV and their impact

The frequency of psychiatric manifestations observed independently of the action of direct HIV infection and the use of psychoactive substances is high in both PLHIV on ARV treatment and PLHIV not yet on treatment [16]. Psychiatric manifestations are a well-identified medical entity and should be investigated in the management of PLHIV, along with the metabolic syndrome, cardiovascular complications, lipodystrophy and other co-morbidities (infections, diabetes, etc.). tuberculosis and hepatitis B and C) [17]. In addition, psychiatric disorders such as anxiety and depression occur in PLHIV undergoing treatment with a therapeutic line containing Efavirenz [19-21]. Indeed, the psychiatric side-effects of the drugs taken by patients must be known and eliminated before attributing psychiatric manifestations to other internal or external causes [21].

Clinically, the spectrum of clinical manifestations is fairly broad and polymorphous without any specificity: cognitive disorders, signs of anxiety, depression and psychosis [1, 2, 13, 16, 17]. The symptoms of depression are not very specific, with an estimated frequency of between 20% and 80%, depending on the series and the population category [6, 12-15]. A number of warning signs should be looked for or taken into account, leading to a diagnosis: these may include asthenia or persistent fatigue with no organic cause, anorexia, sleep disorders, attention problems, feelings of guilt, and recent drug or alcohol addiction in the patient's history [16, 17].

Anxiety may be isolated or associated with depression, which explains why it is so difficult in practice to make a differential diagnosis [6, 17]. Its clinical expression can be quite polymorphous (dry mouth, digestive problems, paresthesia, urticarial eruption, problems concentrating). Its intensity ranges from simple anxiety to a panic attack. The moments of anxiety most often associated with these episodes are the discovery of one's serology, difficulties in sharing one's status with family and friends, therapeutic failure, and a change to a heavier course of treatment [10, 11, 13, 15, 22, 23].

The main psychotic manifestations are manic disorders, hallucinations, delusions and confusion [1, 2, 17, 18]. In the case of hallucinations and persecutory delusions in treatment-experienced PHAs, the adverse effects of Efavirenz should be ruled out [21]. Suicidal ideation and, in particular, suicide attempts should be detected and treated early by specialists. They are more common in women and young MSM, and in people with a psychiatric history [2328].

The problems of stigmatisation and discrimination, patients' failure to accept their serological status, and the guilt of having been infected or of having infected a sexual partner are factors associated with or aggravating psychiatric manifestations in PLHIV, and must be taken into account in the prevention and management of patients suffering from them [10, 29-34]. The consequences of these manifestations may have a negative impact on the individual's socio-professional life (refusal to seek care, loss of motivation and isolation leading to loss of activity or job) or an indirect impact on public health (refusal to take medication with the emergence of resistant sources, refusal to protect oneself during sexual intercourse with an increased risk of transmission for sexual partners).

3. Chemsex and STI/HIV

Chemsex (chemicals used for the enhancement of sexual activitty) is the use of drugs as part of sexual activity. It is a relatively common phenomenon, occurring in between 3% and 29% of men who have sex with men (MSM) [16, 35, 36]. The drugs are of all types (cocaine, amphetamine, etc.) and are used either orally or by injection. Chemsex is often associated with high-risk behaviour for HIV infection and STIs (lack of protection, multiple sexual partners, sexual violence) [35-39].

In addition, chemsex users are often vulnerable because of the effects of psychoactive drugs, with symptoms of aggression, anxiety and sometimes psychotic signs [16, 36].

References

1. Angelino AF, Treisman GJ. Management of psychiatric disorders in patients infected with human immunodeficiency virus Clin Infect Dis 2001;33:847-56.

2. Vlassova N, Angelino AF, Treisman GJ. Update on mental health issues in patients with HIV infection. Curr Infect Dis Rep 2009;11:163-9.

3. Dougherty RH, Skolasky RL Jr, McArthur JC. Progression of HIV-associated dementia treated with HAART. AIDS Read 2002;12:69-74.

4. Chaponda M, Aldhouse N, Kroes M et al. Systematic review of the prevalence of psychiatric illness and sleep disturbance as co-morbidities of HIV infection in the UK. Int J STD AIDS 2018;29:704-713

5. Friedrich F, Aigner M, Fearns N et al. Psychosis in neurosyphilis: clinical aspects and implications Psychopathology 2014;47:3-9.

6. Silvestre D, Linard F, Desi M et al. Anxious-depressive state and cognitive deficit in HIV infection. Encephale 1995; 21:285-8.

7. Friedrich F, Geusau A, Friedrich ME et al. The chameleon of psychiatry - psychiatric manifestations of neurosyphilis. Psychiatr Prax 2012;39:7-13.

8. Parcesepe AM, Mugglin C, Nalugoda F et al. Screening and management of mental health and substance use disorders in HIV treatment settings in low- and middle-income countries within the global IeDEA consortium. J Int AIDS Soc 2018 ;21:e25101. doi: 10.1002/jia2.25101.

9. Corti M. HIV- dementia. A review thirty five years after (1981-2015). Vertex 2015; 26:195201.

10. Bernard C, Dabis F, de Rekeneire N. Prevalence and factors associated with depression in people living with HIV in sub-Saharan Africa: A systematic review and meta-analysis. PLoS One 2017;12:e0181960. doi: 10.1371/journal.pone.0181960. eCollection 2017

11. Treisman G, Angelino A. Interrelation between psychiatric disorders and the prevention and treatment of HIV infection. Clin Infect Dis 2007; 45 (Suppl 4):S313-7

12. Tsai YT, Chen YC, Hsieh CY et al. Incidence of neurological disorders among HIV- infected individuals with universal health care in Taiwan from 2000 to 2010. J Acquir Immune Defic Syndr 2017;75:509-516

13. Kagee A, Martin L. Symptoms of depression and anxiety among a sample of South African patients living with HIV. AIDS Care 2010; 22(2): 159-65.

14. Mateen FJ, Shinohara RT, Carone M et al. Neurologic disorders incidence in HIV+ vs HIV- men: Multicenter AIDS Cohort Study, 1996-2011. Neurology 2012; 79:1873-80.
15. Kagee A, Saal W, Bantjes J. Distress, depression and anxiety among persons seeking HIV testing. AIDS Care 2017;29:280-284.
16. Deike LG, Barreiro P, Reneses B. The new profile of psychiatric disorders in patients with HIV infection. AIDS Rev 2023;25:41-53.
17. Linard F, Jacquemin T. Psychiatric aspects. In Girard MP, Kaltama C, Pialoux G. VIH 2011 Editions Doin 2011
18. McArthur JC. HIV dementia: an evolving disease.J Neuroimmunol 2004; 157:3-10
19. Sumari-de Boer M, Schellekens A, Duinmaijer A et al. Efavirenz is related to neuropsychiatric symptoms among adults, but not among adolescents living with human immunodeficiency virus in Kilimanjaro, Tanzania. Trop Med Int Health 2018;23:164-172
20. Xiao J, Liu Y, Li B et al. Anxiety, depression, and sleep disturbances among people on longterm efavirenz-based treatment for HIV: a cross-sectional study in Beijing, China. BMC Psychiatry 2022;22:710. doi: 10.1186/s12888-022-04366-4.
21. Costa B, Vale N. Efavirenz: History, development and future. Biomolecules 2022 ;13:88. doi: 10.3390/biom13010088
22. Wu YL, Yang HY, Wang J, et al. Prevalence of suicidal ideation and associated factors among HIV-positive MSM in Anhui, China. Int J STD AIDS 2015;26:496-503.
23. Wonde M, Mulat H, Birhanu A et al. The magnitude of suicidal ideation, attempts and associated factors of HIV positive youth attending ART follow ups at St. Paul's hospital Millennium Medical College and St. Peter's specialized hospital, Addis Ababa, Ethiopia, 2018. PLoS One 2019;14:e0224371. doi: 10.1371/journal.pone.0224371. eCollection 2019.
24. Tsegay L, Ayano G. The Prevalence of suicidal ideation and attempt among young people with HIV/AIDS: a systematic review and meta-analysis. Psychiatr 2020;91:1291-1304.
25. Hu FH, Zhao DY, Fu XL et al. Gender differences in suicidal ideation, suicide attempts, and suicide death among people living with HIV: A systematic review and meta-analysis. HIV Med 2023;24:521-532.
26. Necho M, Tsehay M, Zenebe Y. Suicidal ideation, attempt, and its associated factors among HIV/AIDS patients in Africa: a systematic review and meta-analysis study. Int J Ment Health Syst 2021;15:13. doi: 10.1186/s13033-021-00437-3.
27. Tsai YT, Padmalatha S, Ku HC et al. Suicidality among people living with HIV from 2010 to 2021: a systematic review and a meta-regression. Psychosom Med 2022;84:924-939
28. Pei JH, Pei YX, Ma T et al. Prevalence of suicidal ideation, suicide attempt, and suicide plan among HIV/AIDS: A systematic review and meta-analysis.Affect Disord 2021;292:295- 304.
29. Bernard C, Font H, Diallo Z et al. Prevalence and factors associated with severe depressive symptoms in older west African people living with HIV. BMC Psychiatry 2020;20:442. doi: 10.1186/s12888-020-02837-0.
30. Thapinta D, Srithanaviboonchai K, Uthis P et al Association between internalized stigma and depression among people living with HIV in Thailand. Int J Environ Res Public Health. 2022;19:4471. doi: 10.3390/ijerph19084471.
31. Onyebuchi-Iwudibia O, Brown A. HIV and depression in eastern Nigeria: the role of HIV-related stigma. AIDS Care 2014; 26:653-7
32. Kingori C, Reece M, Obeng S et al. Impact of internalized stigma on HIV prevention behaviors among HIV-infected individuals seeking HIV care in Kenya. AIDS Patient Care STDS 2012; 26:761-8.
33. Stahlman S, Grosso A, Ketende S et al. Suicidal ideation among MSM in three West African countries: Associations with stigma and social capital .Int J Soc Psychiatry 2016 ;62:522-31
34. Arashiro P, Maciel CG, Freitas FPR et al. Adherence to antiretroviral therapy in people living with HIV with moderate or severe mental disorder. Sci Rep 2023;13:3569. doi: 10.1038/s41598-

023-30451
35. Nevendorff L, Schroeder SE, Pedrana A et al. Prevalence of sexualized drug use and risk of HIV among sexually active MSM in East and South Asian countries: systematic review and meta-analysis. .J Int AIDS Soc 2023;26:e26054. doi: 10.1002/jia2.26054.
36. Gonzalez-Baeza A, Dolengevich-Segal H, Perez-Valero I et al. Sexualized drug use (Chemsex) is associated with high-risk sexual behaviors and sexually transmitted infections in HIV-positive men who have sex with men: Data from the U-SEX GESIDA 9416 Study. AIDS Patient Care STDS 2018;32:112-118.
37. Maxwell S, Shahmanesh M, Gafos M. Chemsex behaviours among men who have sex with men: A systematic review of the literature. Int J Drug Policy2019; 63:74-89.
38. Ruiz-Robledillo N, Ferrer-Cascales R, Portilla-Tamarit I et al. Chemsex practices and health-related quality of life in spanish men with HIV who have sex with men. .J Clin Med 2021;10:1662. doi: 10.3390/jcm10081662.
39. Guerras JM, Hoyos Miller J, Agusti C et al . Association of sexualized drug use patterns with HIV/STI transmission risk in an internet sample of men who have sex with men from seven European countries. Arch Sex Behav 2021; 50:461-477.

PART VII

VII. 1ST, Sexual health and contraception

Sexually transmitted infections are an integral part of sexual and reproductive health. Sexual health interventions have an impact on STIs, and STIs also have an impact on reproductive health. In the management of 1ST, their interactions with sexual and reproductive health must be known to health professionals and the general population.

1. Impact of STIs on sexual and reproductive health

Most STIs have an impact on the genital tract and can lead to complications. Infections with *Neisseria gonorrheae* and *Chlamydia trachomatis* can cause infertility and sterility in both men and women [1, 2]. Certain STI germs can cause fetopathies (syphilis, zika, herpes), miscarriages or premature deliveries (mycoplasma, chlamydia, gonorrhoea, trichomoniasis) or pelvic inflammatory diseases that are often disabling [3-5]. In addition, some STIs are transmitted from mother to child during pregnancy or childbirth (syphilis, HIV, viral hepatitis B, gonorrhoea, chlamydiosis) [6, 7]. To avoid the impact of these morbidities during the follow-up of pregnant women, systematic screening for certain infections (syphilis, HIV, hepatitis B, genital herpes, chlamydia, gonorrhoea) and their effective and appropriate management is planned [7]. Throughout pregnancy, pregnant women should be screened for symptomatic or asymptomatic STIs. Screening can be repeated if there is a positive assessment of the woman's risk of exposure to STIs (the sexual partner's high-risk behaviour may expose the woman to STIs and HIV throughout pregnancy). Pregnancy may also be the cause of the recurrence of certain STIs, such as genital herpes, genital candidiasis or the clinical expression of genital warts or the discovery of cervical dysplasia due to HPV infection.

2. STIs and contraception

Most family planning methods do not protect against STIs [8]. But the interactions between contraception and STIs depend largely on risky sexual behaviour. One of the markers between STIs and contraception in young people is the frequency with which unwanted pregnancies occur. In young people, only the correct and systematic use of condoms provides effective protection against STIs and unwanted pregnancies; this is why we talk of dual protection [9, 10].

Certain contraceptive methods have an impact on the occurrence of certain infections (although these are not true STIs). Vaginal candidiasis is more common in women using oral contraceptives [11], and bacterial vaginosis is more common in women using diaphragms with spermicides [12]. In addition, repeated high-dose use of spermicide is associated with an increased risk of genital lesions, which increases the risk of contracting HIV infection. This is why this method is not recommended for women at high risk of HIV infection or those who are already infected [13].

Method	Effectiveness in preventing pregnancy	Protection against 1ST
Male condom	85-98 %	Protects against most 1ST and HIV Unproven protection against 1ST transmitted by skin contact (herpes, HPV, scabiosis, pediculosis, monkeypox)
Female condom	79-95 %	Protects against 1ST and HIV in women Further studies needed in men
Spermicide	71-85 %	Possible protection against 1ST bacteria No protection against 1ST viruses May increase the risk of HIV infection
Diaphragm with spermicide	84-94 %	Possible protection against 1ST bacteria No protection against 1ST viruses, in particular HIV, but does protect against cervical neoplasia Increases the risk of bacterial vaginosis May increase the risk of HIV infection
Oral	92-99 %	No protection against 1ST and lower genital tract infections

contraceptives		Increases the frequency of candidiasis Reducing the risk of symptomatic pelvic inflammatory disease
Implants	> 99 %	No protection against 1ST and HIV
Injections	> 99 %	No protection against 1ST and lower genital tract infections Reducing the risk of symptomatic pelvic inflammatory disease
Intrauterine device (IUD)	> 99 %	No protection against 1ST Associated with an increased risk of symptomatic pelvic inflammatory syndrome
Surgical sterilisation (tubal ligation and vasectomy)	> 99 %	No protection against STIs No protection against lower genital tract infections Reducing the risk of symptomatic pelvic inflammatory disease

Table 14: Contraceptive methods: effectiveness in preventing pregnancy and sexually transmitted infections [14].

References

1. Tsevat DG, Wiesenfeld HC, C et al Sexually transmitted diseases and infertility. Am J Obstet Gynecol 2017; 16:1-9.

2. Pellati D, Mylonakis I, Bertolon G et al. Genital tract infections and infertility Eur J Obstet Gynecol Reprod Biol 2008;140:3-11.

3. Moodley P, A W Sturm AW. Sexually transmitted infections, adverse pregnancy outcome and neonatal infection. Semin Neonatol 2000;5:255-69.

4. Lemly D, Gupta N. Sexually Transmitted Infections Part 2: Discharge Syndromes and Pelvic Inflammatory Disease. Pediatr Rev 2020;41:522-537.

5. Shroff S. Infectious Vaginitis, Cervicitis, and Pelvic Inflammatory Disease. Med Clin North Am 2023;107:299-315.

6. Rowley J, Vander-hoom S, Korenromp E et al. Chlamydia, gonorrheae, trichomiasis and syphilis. Global prevalence and incidence estimates. Bull Word health Organ 2019; 97: 548562

7. Moreira J, Peisoto TM, Siquiera AM et al. Sexually acquired Zika virus: a systematic review. Clin Microbiol Infect 2017; 23 :296-305

8. McGregor JA, Hammill HA. Contraception and sexually transmitted diseases: interactions and opportunities. Am J Obstet Gynecol 1993;168:2033-41.

9. Raidoo S, Kaneshiro B. Contraception counseling for adolescents. Curr Opin Obstet Gynecol. 2017;29:310-315

10. Steiner RJ, Pampati S, Kortsmit KM et al. Long-acting reversible contraception, condom use, and sexually transmitted infections: A systematic review and meta-analysis. Am J Prev Med 2021;61:750-760.

11. Overton ET, Shacham E, Singhatiraj E et al. Incidence of sexually transmitted infections among HIV-infected women using depot medroxyprogesterone acetate contraception. Contraception 2008;78:125-30

12. d'Oro LC, Parazzini F, Naldi L et al. Barrier methods of contraception, spermicides, and sexually transmitted diseases: a review. Genitourin Med 1994 ;70:410-7.

13. Morrison CS, Turner AN, Jones LB. Highly effective contraception and acquisition of HIV and other sexually transmitted infections. Best Pract Res Clin Obstet Gynaecol 2009;23:263- 84.

14. World Health Organisation (WHO). Sexually transmitted infections and other reproductive tract infections. Essential practices guide. Geneva 2005

PART VIII

VIII. Prevention and screening for 1ST and HIV

1. Prevention

When treating patients suffering from STIs, the prescription of treatment should be accompanied by prevention advice based on information about 1STs and HIV [1, 2]. In practice, the diagnosis of an STI is proof that the patient has engaged in sexual behaviour that puts them at risk of contracting 1ST and that they have not yet learned the prevention messages [1].

The consultation should be used as an opportunity to pass on personalised messages and encourage patients to adopt responsible, low-risk sexuality by helping them to change their behaviour. Individual, confidential communication should provide the patient with knowledge of the routes of contamination, the means of prevention and the potential consequences of STIs for him and his partner(s) (infertility, cervical cancer and human papilloma virus infection, hepatocellular carcinoma and hepatitis B, risk of contracting HIV infection with all its morbidity). An important element in communication is to avoid making patients feel guilty or judging them.

The importance and benefits of systematically using condoms for all sexual relations outside the context of a stable couple must be stressed. As well as wearing a condom, the patient should be encouraged to reduce the number of sexual partners. Patients should be told of the need and importance of taking care of their partner(s) in order to break the chain of transmission and, above all, avoid the complications associated with untreated STIs. Treatment must be properly explained to facilitate compliance, which is the key to its effectiveness. During treatment, sexual abstinence or protected intercourse is recommended to avoid contaminating sexual partners and cut the chain of transmission. The follow-up visit enables the efficacy of the treatment to be checked and the patient to resume his or her normal sex life, adopting safer behaviour.

Strategies to prevent HIV infection involve communication to change individual and collective behaviour, and promoting the use of condoms [3, 4]. Biomedical interventions have been shown to be effective, such as prevention of mother-to-child transmission (effective treatment with antiretroviral tritherapies), pre-exposure prophylaxis (PrEP) and post-exposure prophylaxis with ARV drugs [4-9]. In Africa, male circumcision has been proposed in high-prevalence countries as a strategy for preventing HIV in men [11,12]. Prevention of mosquito bites (mosquito nets, insecticides) and the destruction of larval habitats are effective strategies in the event of a Zika virus epidemic.

HPV vaccination should be offered to all adolescents (girls and boys) after the age of 10 [13]. There is considerable scientific evidence not only of effective prevention of HIV-induced cancer in vaccinated women, but also of a significant reduction in HPV infections in boys and girls who have received the vaccine [14]. Hepatitis B vaccination should be offered at birth to all children and adults who have had no contact with the virus [15]. In the event of an Ebola epidemic, there is an effective vaccine that targets the populations to be vaccinated (healthcare professionals, people exposed in the endemic zone). The vaccine against monkeypox is also effective, and is recommended as a priority for high-risk populations such as MSM.

2. Screening

To prevent and better control 1ST, most countries have defined a screening strategy targeting at-risk individuals and certain vulnerable groups [2, 16].

Patient suffering from an STI

Screening for HIV, syphilis, hepatitis B and hepatitis C should be systematically offered to patients suffering from an STI [16].

Sexual partners of a patient suffering from an STI

To cut the chain of transmission of STIs, it is recommended that all sexual partners of symptomatic patients be treated. In this context, screening for other STIs should be offered as a matter of course: gonorrhoea, chlamydia, syphilis, HIV, hepatitis B and, depending on the case, hepatitis C [2,16]. Systematic screening for certain STIs such as herpes, trichomoniasis and candidiasis does not contribute and has no added value either individually or in terms of public health [2].

Pregnant woman

Given that the majority of STIs can be transmitted from mother to child, and that the hormonal and immunological background favours the recurrence of certain STIs, it is recommended that routine screening be offered for HIV, syphilis, hepatitis B (in the absence of vaccination), gonococcal disease and chlymadiosis [2]. During antenatal visits, attention should be paid to detecting a growth (or recurrence) of genital herpes and the appearance of condylomata and cervical dysplasia. The possibility of screening for hepatitis C should be discussed on a case-by-case basis if there is a risk of exposure (IV drug use, tattooing; iterative blood transfusion) [16].

Men who have sex with men (MSM)

In this group, given the risk involved, screening for HIV, syphilis, hepatitis B and C, gonorrhoea and chlamydia should be offered as a matter of course, with anal and oral swabs taken [2]. You should also be screened for HPV and anal cancer.

Teenagers

In practice, screening can be offered to adolescents with multiple partners who do not use condoms regularly, and to those with a personal history of chlamydial infection or a history of infection in a partner. Screening should be offered for HIV, gonorrhoea, chlamydia and syphilis [2].

People who have suffered sexual abuse

Where sexual abuse is suspected (or known), screening for STIs should be systematic (and may be medico-legal) for both the person exposed to the abuse and the presumed perpetrator [2, 17-19]: HIV, syphilis, hepatitis B and C, gonorrhoea, chlamydia. Serological monitoring of certain infections such as HIV and syphilis is recommended in order to document subsequent seropositivity due to this exposure.

Reference

1. Derancourt C, Vernay-Vaisse C, Spenatto N et al. Prevention of STD/STIs. Ann Dermatol Venereol 2016; 143: 786-791
2. Centers for Diseases Control and Prevention. Sexually transmitted infections treatement. Guidelines 2021. MMR 2021; 70: 30-59
3. Kurth AE, Celum C, Baeten JM et al. Combination HIV prevention: significance, challenges, and opportunities. Curr HIV/AIDS Rep 2011;8:62-72.
4. Baeten JM, Donnell D, Ndase P et al Antiretroviral prophylaxis for HIV prevention in heterosexual men and women. .N Engl J Med. 2012;367:399-410.
5. Phanuphak N, Gulick RM. HIV treatment and prevention 2019: current standards of care. Curr Opin HIV AIDS. 2020;15:4-12.
6. Engelman KD, Engelman AN. Long-acting cabotegravir for HIV/AIDS prophylaxis. Biochemistry 2021;60:1731-1740
7. Molina JM, Ghosn J, Assoumou L et al. Daily and on-demand HIV pre-exposure prophylaxis with emtricitabine and tenofovir disoproxil (ANRS PREVENIR): a prospective observational cohort study. Lancet HIV 2022;9:e554-e562. doi: 10.1016/S2352-3018(22)00133-3
8. Laurent C, Dembele Keita B, Yaya I et al. HIV pre-exposure prophylaxis for men who have sex with men in west Africa: a multicountry demonstration study. Lancet HIV 2021;8:e420- e428. doi: 10.1016/S2352-3018(21)00005-9.
9. Yap PK, Loo Xin GL, Tan YY et al. Antiretroviral agents in pre-exposure prophylaxis: emerging and advanced trends in HIV prevention. J Pharm Pharmacol 2019 ;71:1339-1352.
10. Khanna AS, Roberts ST, Cassels S et al. Estimating PMTCT's impact on heterosexual HIV transmission: a mathematical modeling analysis. PLoS One 2015;10:e0134271. doi:

10.1371/journal.pone.0134271.
11. Njeuhmeli E, Hatzold K, Gold E et al. Lessons learned from scale-up of voluntary medical male circumcision focusing on adolescents: benefits, challenges, and potential opportunities for linkages with adolescent HIV, sexual, and reproductive health services. J Acquir Immune Defic Syndr2014; 66 (Suppl 2):S193-9.
12. SK, Reed JB, Thomas A et al. Achieving the HIV prevention impact of voluntary medical male circumcision: lessons and challenges for managing programmes. PLoS Med 2014;11:e1001641. doi: 10.1371/journal.pmed.1001641.
13. Lei J, Ploner A, Elfstrom M et al. HPV vaccine and risk on invasive cervical cancer. N Engl J Med 2020 ;383 :1340-8
14. Basu P, Malvi SG, Joshi S et al. Vaccine efficacy persistent HPV 16/18 infection at 10 years after one, two and tree doses of quadrivalent HPV vaccine in gils in India: multicentre prospective cohort study. Lancet Oncol 2021; 22 :1518-29
15. Le Turnier P, Charreau I, Gabassi A et al. Hepatitis A and B vaccine uptake and immunisation among men who have sex with men seeking PrEP: a substudy of the ANRS IPERGAY trial. Sex Transm Infect 2023; 99:140-142.
16. Vernay-Vaisse C, Spenatto N, Derancourt C et al. STD/STI screening. Ann Dermatol Venereol 2016; 143: 703-09
17. Pitche P, Kombate K, Gbadoe AD et al. Sexually transmitted diseases in young children in Lome (Togo). Role of sexual abuse. Arch Pediatr 2001; 8:25-31
18. Greenberg JB. Childhood sexual abuse and sexually transmitted diseases in adults: a review of and implications for STD/HIV programmes. Int J STD AIDS 2001;12:777-83
19. Driscoll SJ, Fidler KJ, Shears A et al Sexually transmitted infections in suspected child sexual abuse. Arch Dis Child2023;108:53-55.
20. Qin X, Melvin AJ. Laboratory Diagnosis of Sexually Transmitted Infections in Cases of Suspected Child Sexual Abuse. J Clin Microbiol 2020;58:e01433-19. doi: 10.1128/JCM.01433-19.

Iconography

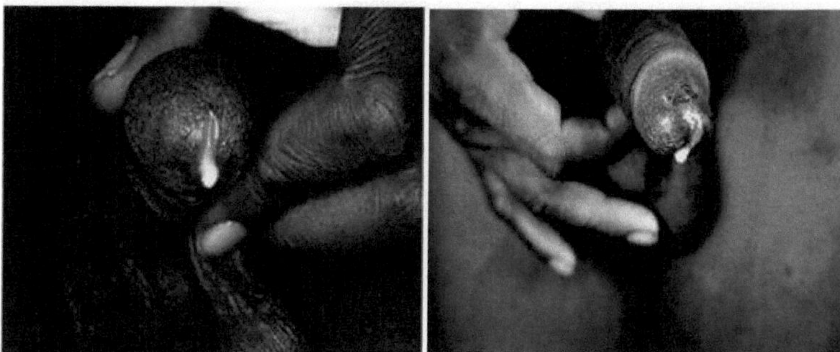

Figure 7: Gonococcal urethritis Figure 8: Gonococcal urethritis

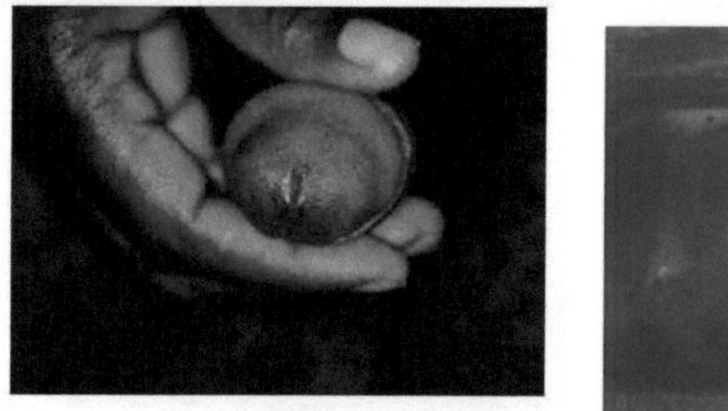

Figure 9: Chlamydial urethritis Figure 10: Chlamydial cervicitis

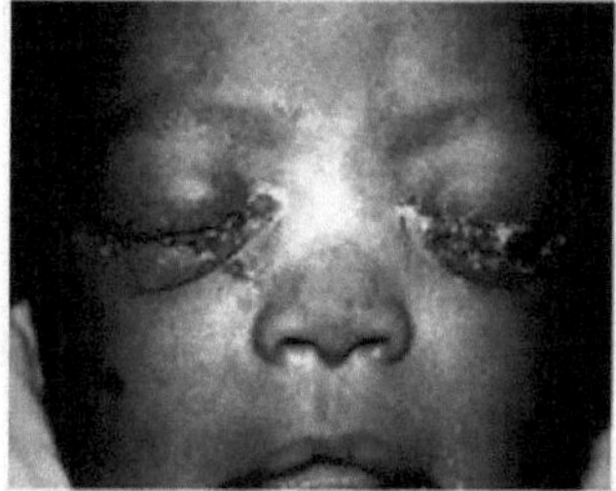

Figure 11: Gonococcal conjunctivitis

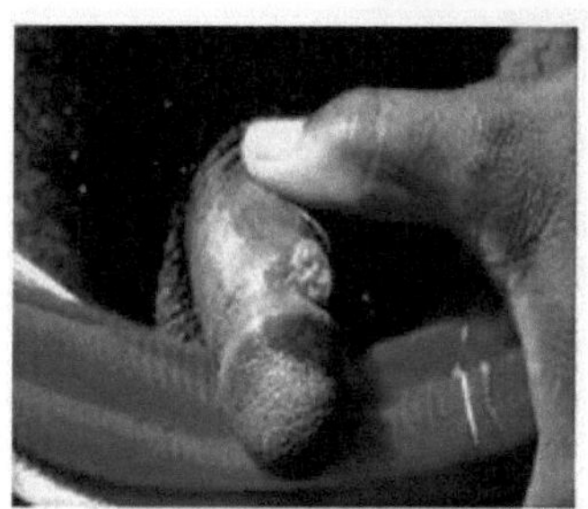

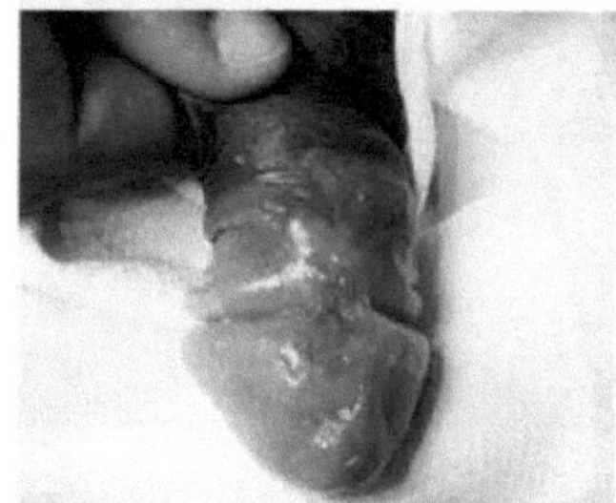

Figure 12: Syphilitic canker Figure 13: Syphilitic canker

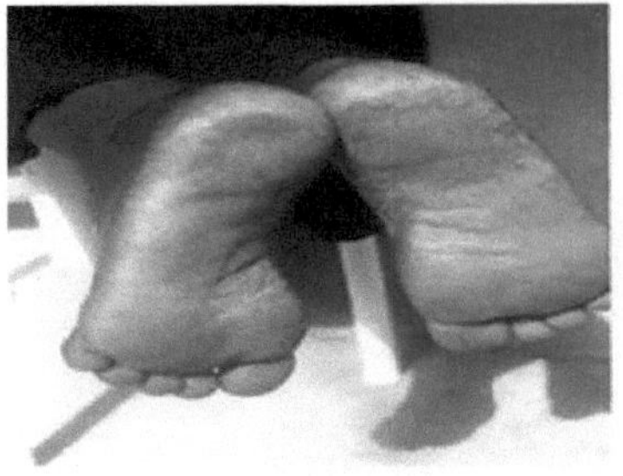
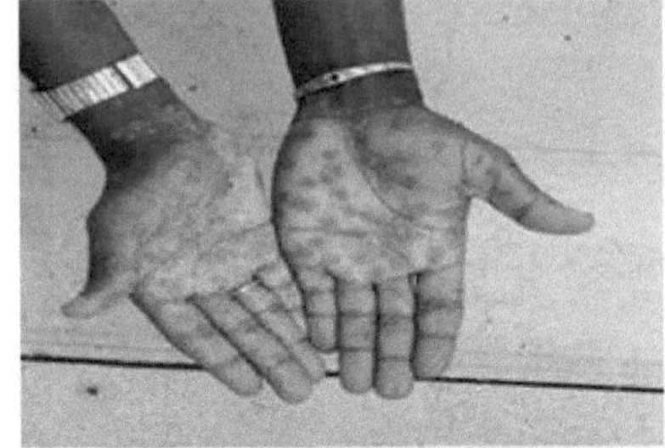

Figure 14: Plantar syphilis Figure 15: Palmar syphilis

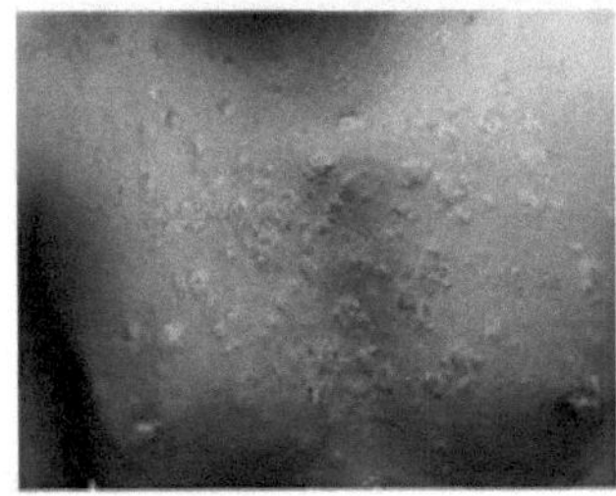
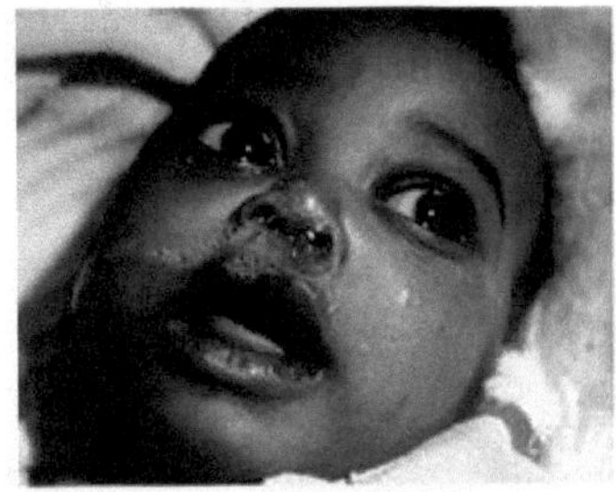

Figure 16: Syphilis of the trunk Figure 17: Congenital syphilis: Coryza

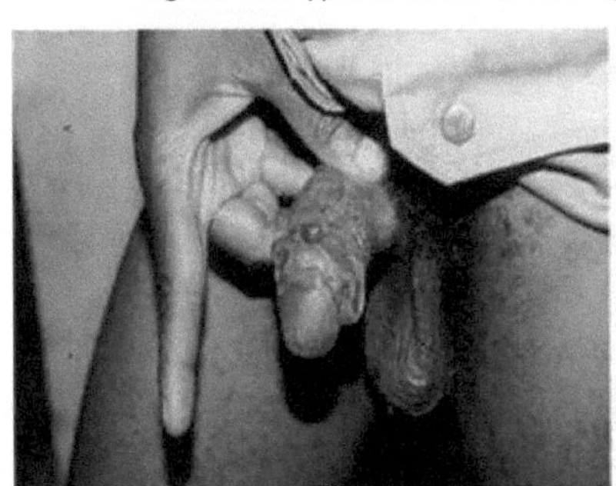
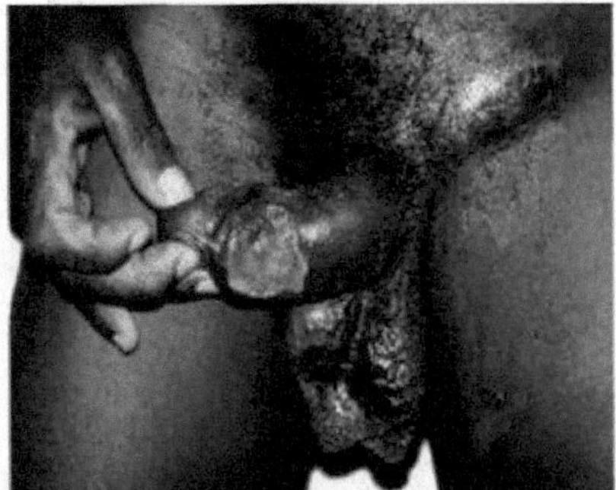

Figure 18: Soft canker (multiple ulcerations) Figure 19: Soft canker (deep ulceration)

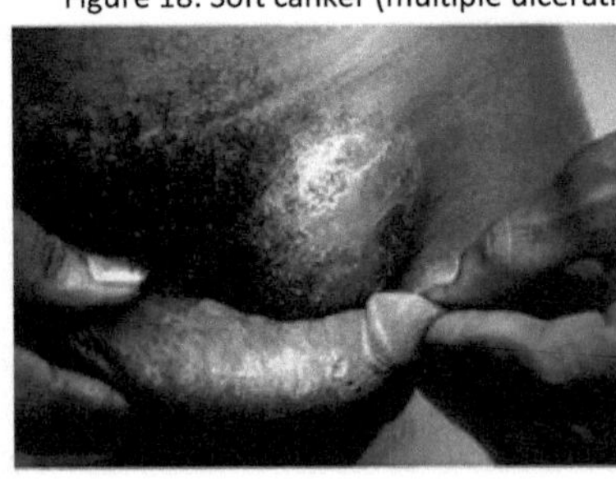
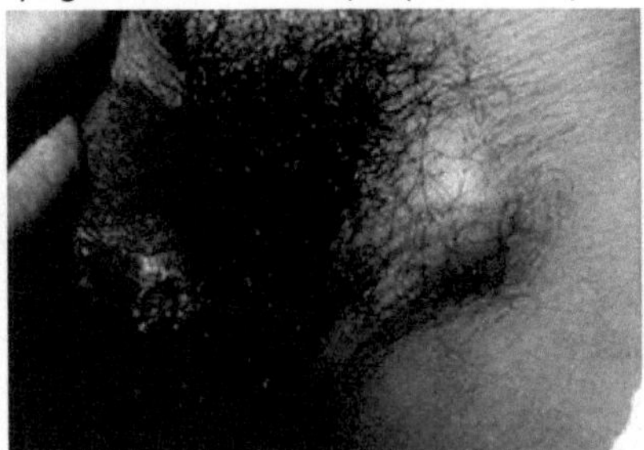

Figure 20: Soft canker: ulceration and inguinal bubo Figure 21: Soft canker: ulceration and inguinal bubo

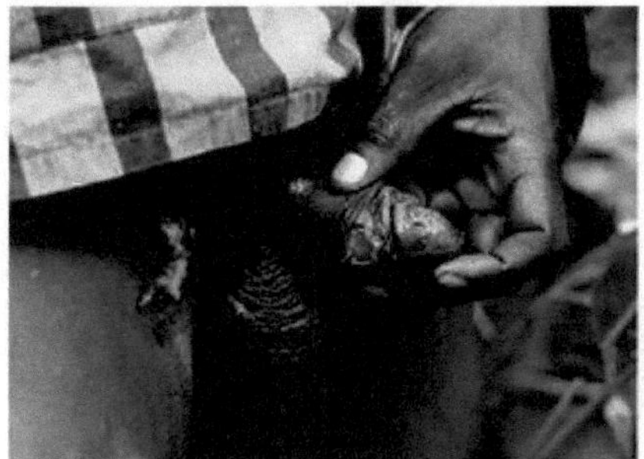

Figure 22: Soft canker: ulceration and inguinal bubo

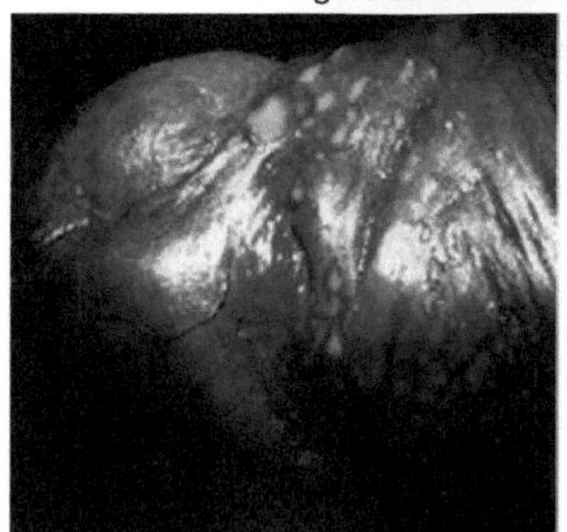

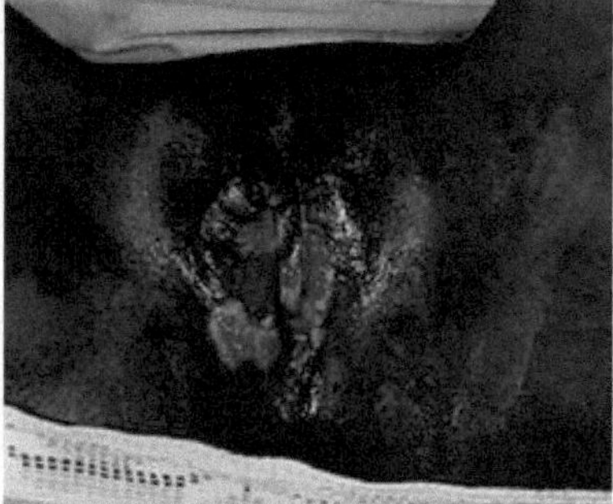

Figure 23: Genital herpes Figure 24: Genital herpes

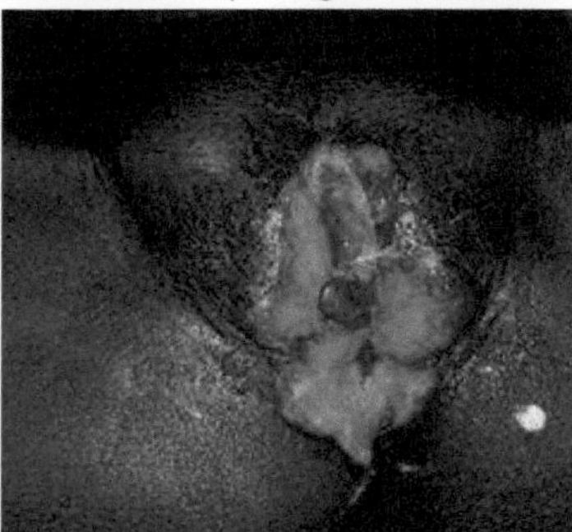

Figure 25: Giant and chronic herpes in HIV patients

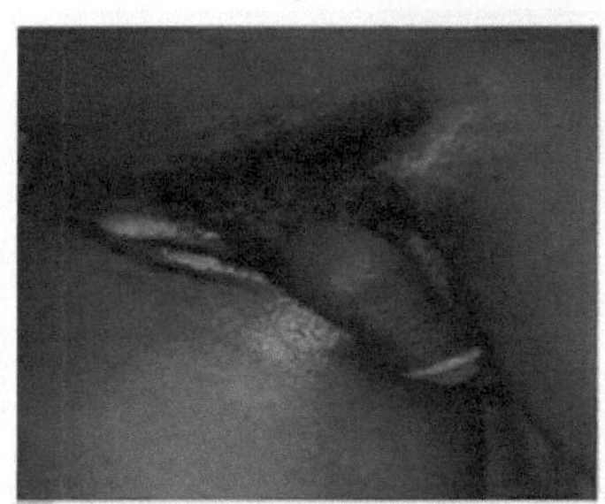

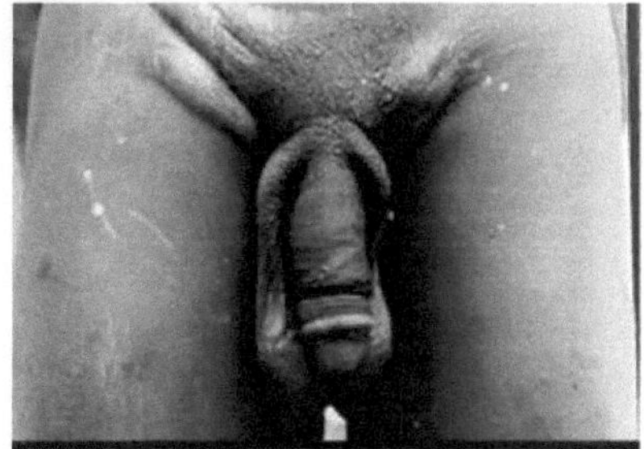

Fig. 26 and 27: Lymphogranulomatosis venereum: oblong adenopathies with Poulie's sign

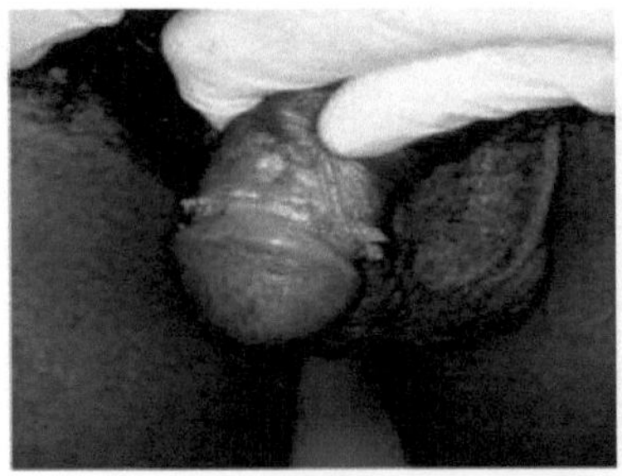

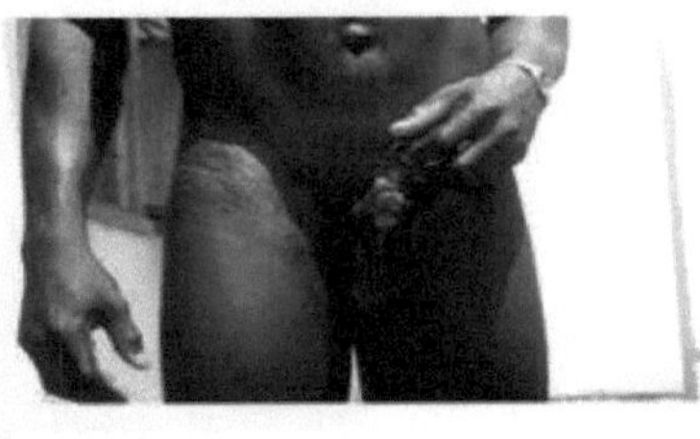

Figure 26: Condylomata Figure 27: Condylomata

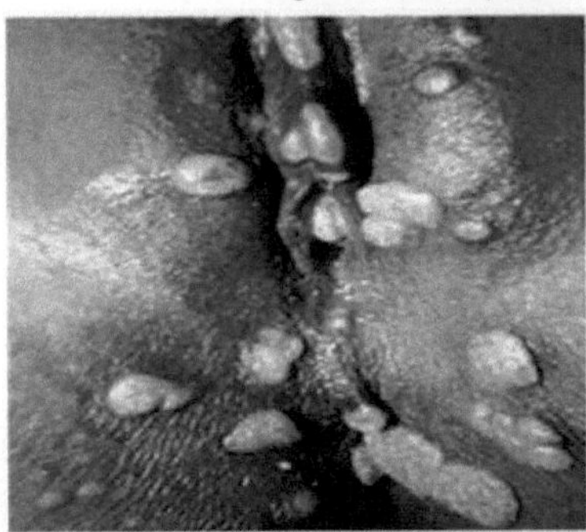

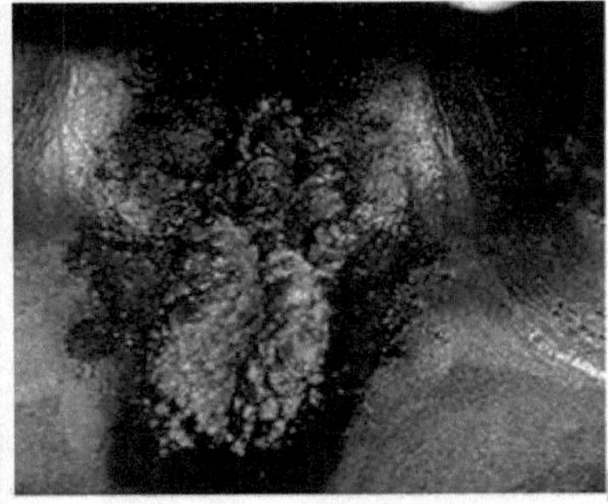

Figure 28 Vulvar and perineal condylomata Figure 29: Vulvar condylomata

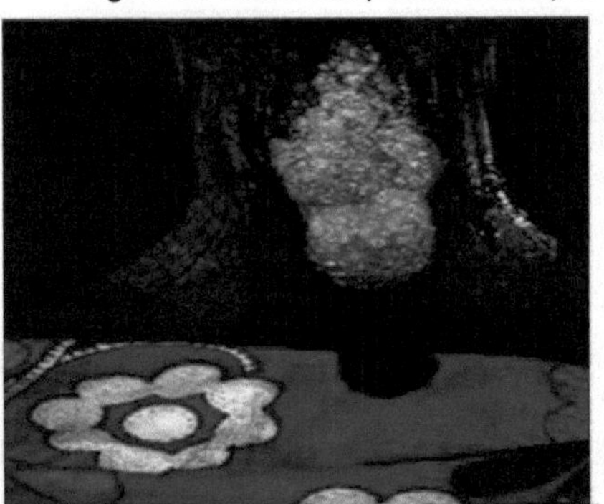

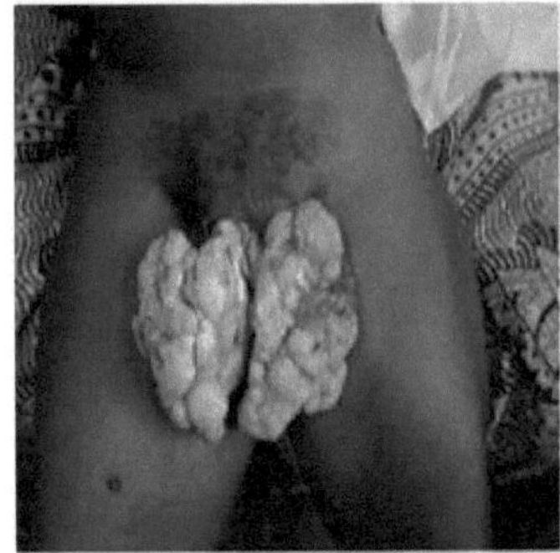

Figure 30: Giant condyloma (Buske's tumour) Figure 31: Giant condyloma (Buske's tumour)

PART IX

IX. Syndromic management of STIs

1. Rationale for syndromic management

In developing countries, particularly in Africa, given the limited technical resources available and the scarcity of qualified health workers, syndromic management has become the norm, particularly in most peripheral health centres. Syndromic management of STIs has been recommended and supported by the WHO as part of HIV and AIDS programmes for countries with limited resources [1, 2]. This approach has made it possible to decentralise STI treatment within the framework of task delegation (training of medical and paramedical staff based on algorithms with guides containing standardised therapeutic protocols) [2-5].

The syndromic management process is well defined: based on epidemiological studies carried out in most countries, and taking into account the morbidity of certain germs, treatments are directed according to the clinical syndrome adapted to the patient's sex. We know that in men, N. gonorrheae and C. trachomatis are the most frequent and most morbid germs in urethritis [3-8]. In practice, when urethritis occurs in men, these two germs should be treated at the same time. In women, the main causes of vaginitis are Trichomonas vaginalis, Candidas albicans and Gardnerella vaginalis, while N. gonorrheae and C. trachomatis are the main causes of cervicitis. Therapeutic management should take these factors into account, in order to be more effective in the management of STIs in women [5-8]. In the case of leucorrhoea, the two causes of cervicitis or, in the absence of risk factors for STIs, vaginitis should be treated simultaneously as a matter of priority. In the case of genital ulceration, whatever the sex, syphilis and genital herpes (and possibly chancroid, depending on the epidemiological context) should be treated first [7].

The syndromic approach has a number of drawbacks: it only targets symptomatic cases, with a tendency to underestimate asymptomatic infections, particularly in women and sexual partners [10-12]. This is why it is currently recommended as part of health programmes for certain vulnerable populations to offer etiological diagnosis using rapid test kits [13-15]. In practice, however, in countries with limited resources, these tests are not available everywhere, which is why the syndromic approach is still used in these countries, particularly in the majority of peripheral health centres, in order to bring care closer to patients (geographical accessibility of care).

2. Overview of approaches to the management of STIs in practice

In medical practice, there are three approaches to disease management:

- *Etiological approach.* Laboratory tests are used to identify the infectious agent. This is the most precise method; it requires substantial resources (human resources and adequate technical facilities) and financial costs for the patient (consultation and paraclinical diagnostic costs).
- *Clinical approach without laboratory examination.* It is based on clinical judgement and is the least reliable of the methods. It depends too much on the experience and expertise of specialist doctors and is not effective in general and peripheral healthcare centres.
- Syndromic management. This is the management of patients presenting with a set of symptoms and clinical signs compatible with different 1ST for all the infectious agents involved in the etiology of these clinical symptoms.

In practice, each approach has advantages and disadvantages that need to be **understood.**

Table 15: Advantages and disadvantages of diagnostic approaches

TYPES OF APPROACH	BENEFITS	DISADVANTAGES
CLINIC	- Rapid relief - Can be applied anywhere - Not dependent on Laboratory	- Frequent diagnostic errors - Encourages resistance - Does not support associations - Requires a high level of

		professional expertise
ETIOLOGY	- Reliability and precision - Enables treatment germ-specific - Prevents resistance - Takes into account associations - Better monitoring	- Time-consuming - Laboratory required team - Accessibility not always guarantees (financial and geographic) for patients - High cost - Reliability of results varies according to the level of technical facilities available
SYNDROMIQUE	- Support for associations - Time savings - No risk of patient loss - Increases the chances of recovery - Can be applied anywhere - Easy to apply	- Does not include asymptomatic patients - Risk of treatment with exces - Not accepted by all care providers - Notification problem partners

3. The different stages of the syndromic approach [6].

The syndromic approach in practice involves several stages
- Reception and physical examination
- Diagnosis and correct treatment of symptomatic STIs,
- Taking care of partners
- The Board

This approach must be rigorous and taught to all healthcare providers involved in the syndromic management of STIs in order to guarantee the quality of services delivered to patients, whatever the centre.

Reception and physical examination

► *The reception* is the first stage, the first contact with the patient. It enables a climate of trust to be established between the healthcare staff and the patient, and the interview to be undertaken in a calm atmosphere. It's important to understand from the outset that interviewing a person suffering from an STI is a special process. This is because the symptoms are located in the genital area, which causes patients to feel a certain amount of embarrassment. Patients may hide this essential information from the clinician, or find it difficult to answer accurately. So, in order to question patients effectively, you need to gain their trust quickly (from the first contact) if you want to gather valuable information in the short time you have available in the consultation.

Attitudes and certain gestures are useful in winning the trust of your patients
- Welcome your patients when they arrive in the consultation room;
- Look at them when you ask them questions;
- Emphasise the private and confidential nature of the consultation.

Attitudes that can cause genetics in patients and should be avoided
- Don't say hello when he arrives at the surgery;
- Don't look at him when you ask him questions;
- Use an accusatory tone;
- Use unintelligible vocabulary ;
- Receive two patients at a time in the office or consultation room;
- Reading papers or magazines during consultation ;
- Display an unfriendly expression during the consultation.

All these precautions do not take up any extra time, but rather help to ensure that patients are well received, that their confidence is gained and that they can be effectively questioned.

► *Questioning is* an important part of the syndromic management of STIs. It should be relaxed but rigorous and should include the following steps.

General questions: age, marital status, occupation of the patient and his/her partner, number of children, whether the patient is travelling or away from home.

Reason for consultation: identify the symptoms or complaints that prompted the consultation and their duration.

Risk factor screening: This should be compulsory and systematically carried out in the search for key information about sexual history and risky sexual behaviour.

- personal sexual history (number of partners in the year, type of partners, new partners in the last three months, partner with or who has had an STI, whether or not condoms were used);
- sexual behaviour of the STI-infected partner; number of partners
- alcohol consumption and drug use by the patient and/or his/her partner(s).

Medical history: it is important to check for the existence of a previous STI and any allergies to certain drugs.

Physical examination

The physical examination is used to confirm or refute the patient's complaints. The physical examination is compulsory, systematic and fairly exhaustive; it must be loco-regional and general in good conditions of confidentiality and illumination.

► *Chez rhomme.*

Examination of the penis: look for ulcers (sores); urethral discharge (massage the urethra to check for the presence or absence of discharge); tumours (vegetations or condylomas). If the patient is not circumcised, the prepuce should be removed and the glans, preputial groove and urethral meat examined.

Examination of the scrotum: the scrotum should be palpated to try to detect any abnormalities of the testicles, epididymis and spermatic cord.

Examination of the oral cavity: look for sores, oral candidiasis, tumours or pharyngitis.

Examination of lymph nodes for inguinal adenopathy (inguinal bubo) or generalized adenopathy (AIDS).

Examination of the anus: look for sores, condylomata and discharge.

Skin examination: look for eruptions and ulcerations and examine the palms of the hands and soles of the feet.

► *In women*

Examination of the vagina and cervix. This is carried out using a speculum, which is carefully inserted into the vagina to look for any discharge, lesions or growths in the vagina or cervix.

Bimanual examination (vaginal touch with abdominal palpation). Carefully and delicately, the vaginal walls, cervix and surrounding areas should be palpated for upper genital pain, which may suggest pelvic inflammatory disease. Urethral discharge can be demonstrated by scraping the upper part of the vagina from back to front with the intravaginal finger and applying pressure to the pelvis with the abdominal hand. The lower abdomen should be examined systematically, looking for pain, resistance (defensiveness) or a mass when the abdomen is palpated.

Examination of the perineum and vulva. The perineum and vulva should be examined for discharge (white discharge), ulcers and tumours (condylomas).

Examination of the anus: this should be carried out systematically and may reveal ulcers, condylomata or pus discharge.

Examination of the oral cavity: This is used to check for sores, candidiasis, tumours and pharyngitis.

Examination of lymph nodes: look for inguinal adenopathy or generalized adenopathy;

Skin examination: Looking for wounds and rashes;

4. The main STI syndromes

Table 16: Clinical characteristics and causes of 1ST syndromes

SYNDROMES	SYMPTOMS (complaints)	SIGNS	ETIOLOGIES
Urethral discharge	- Purulent or serous discharge - Burning while urinating - Tingling of the urethral meat	- Urethral discharge	-*Neisseria gonorrhoeae* (Gonorrhoea) -*Chlamydia trachomatis* (Chlamydiasis) - *Mycoplasma hominis* (Mycoplasma) -*Trichomonas vaginalis* (Trichomoniasis)
Vaginal discharge	- Mucopurulent vaginal discharge - Pain on urination - Pruritus or itching - Pelvic pain - Pain during sexual intercourse (dyspareunia)	- Vaginal discharge (Leucorrhea) or not - Vulvar irritation -Cervicitis with or without discharge	-*Neisseria gonorrhoeae* (Gonorrhoea) - *Chlamydia trachomatis* (Chlamydiasis) -*Trichomonas vaginalis* (Trichomoniasis) -*Candidas albicans* (Candidiasis) - *Gardnerella vaginalis* (gardenellosis)
Lower abdominal pain	- Lower abdominal or pelvic pain - Mucopurulent vaginal discharge	- Pelvic pain on gynaecological examination and/or - Vaginal discharge - Cervicitis	-*Neisseria gonorrhoeae* (Gonorrhoea) -*Chlamydia trachomatis* (Chlamydiasis
Genital ulceration	Genital wound	- Genital ulceration -Vesicles	-*Treponema pallidum* (Syphilis) -*Haemophilus ducreyi* (soft canker) -*Herpes simplex virus* (genital herpes)
Inguinal bubo	Painful inguinal tumefaction	- Painful unilateral or bilateral adenopathy(ies) - Genital or non-genital ulceration	-*Chlamydia trachomatis* (Chlamydiasis) -*Haemophilus ducreyi* (soft canker)
Tumour of the scrotum	Pain and/or Tumour of the scrotum	-Pain and/or -Tumour of the scrotum	-*Neisseria gonoeahoeae* (Gonococcal disease) -*Chlamydia trachomatis* (Chlamydia)
Conjontivitis in newborns	- Purulent secretions from an eye or ear - Eye Rodent - Tumefaction of the eyelids.	- Purulent discharge - Conjunctival rodent - eyelid edema	-*Neisseria gonorrhoeae* (Gonorrhoea) -*Chlamydia trachomatis* (Chlamydiasis)
Condylomata or venereal vegetation	-Growths or cocksucking	- Painless, irregular excrescences, with or without pedicles	- *Human Papilloma Virus* HPV (condyloma)

Several scientific and operational evaluations of these syndromes have made it possible to assess their sensitivity and specificity in clinical practice [8, 9, 16-19]. Some syndromes, such as urethral discharge and genital ulceration, have good sensitivity and specificity; on the other hand, the sensitivity and specificity of the vaginal discharge and lower abdominal pain syndromes are fairly low, with a significant underestimation of asymptomatic cases, hence the current promotion of rapid etiological screening tests in women (and adolescents) and in certain vulnerable groups such as sex workers and men who have sex with men [20, 21]. It is important to emphasise that the syndromic approach is a diagnostic tool for symptomatic cases, ***but is not at all a tool to be used for 1ST screening*** [17].

5. Diagnosis and treatment of different syndromes

Urethral discharge

Urethral discharge is the flow of a liquid abnormal in appearance, odour or abundance through the urethra.

Clinical characteristics

The appearance of urethral discharge varies. It may be purulent (whitish or greenish-yellow) or serous (transparent). Abundance ranges from a clear discharge to small stains on linen, pressure on the urethra, or even just a crust on the urethral meat observed in the morning during the first micturition. The discharge may be accompanied by burning and tingling of the urethral fluid.

Causes

- Frequent and morbid causes: *Neisseria gonorrhoeae* (Gonorrhoea) *Chlamydia trachomatis* (Chlamydiosis)
- Less frequent and less morbid causes: *Trichomonas vaginalis* (Trichomoniasis); *Mycoplasma genitalium,*

In practice, the clinical appearance of the discharge does not allow it to be linked to a specific germ. Several germs are often associated with the same discharge (mixed cause).

Treatment

- Patients presenting with urethral discharge should be treated at the same time, from the first consultation, for: gonorrhoea, chlamydia, etc.
- If symptoms persist, despite good compliance, patients should be treated for trichomoniasis.

Figure 32: Urethral discharge algorithm

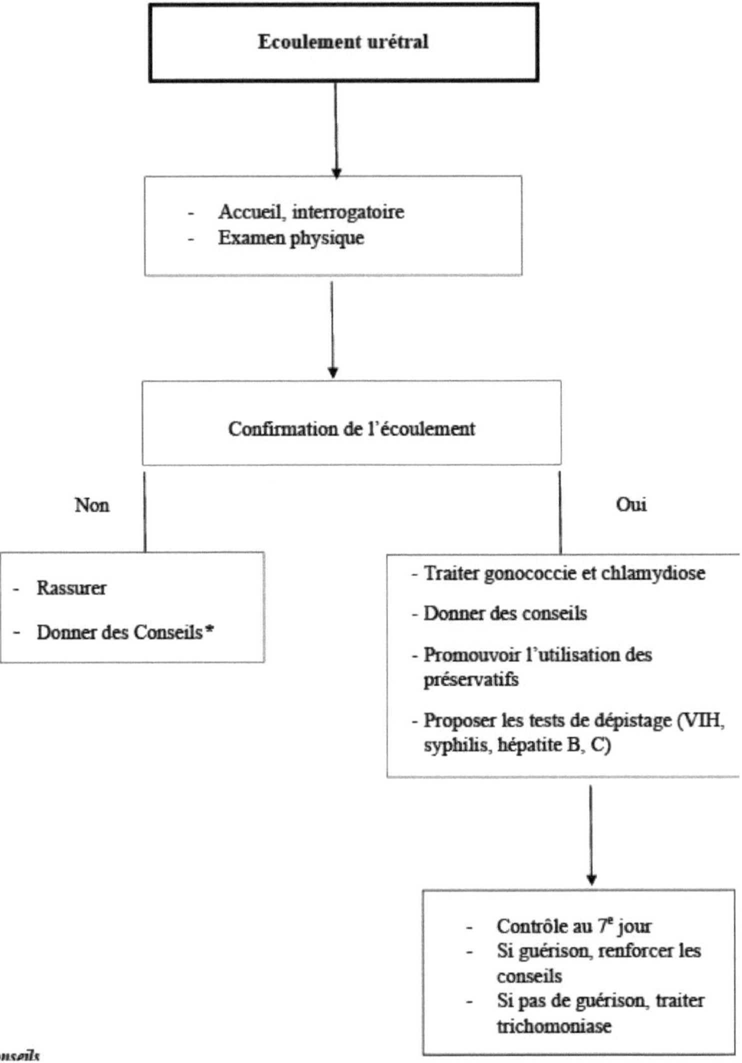

- Information on the means of transmission and prevention of 1ST
- Promoting low-risk behaviour
- Promoting the use of condoms

Vaginal discharge

In women, there is usually a "normal" vaginal discharge or physiological discharge. The discharge becomes abnormal in odour, abundance or appearance.

Clinical characteristics

Vaginal discharge may be accompanied by vulvar irritation, itching, pain on urination, pelvic pain or dyspareunia (pain during intercourse). It may be vaginitis, cervicitis or cervico-vaginitis.

Cervicitis has few symptoms. However, it may consist of mucopurulent vaginal discharge associated with pelvic pain. However, cervicitis is often asymptomatic.

Vaginitis is characterised by abnormal vaginal discharge, often abundant and sometimes malodorous, with or without itching. These symptoms are not specific to one germ, and the three germs responsible for vaginitis may present with the same symptoms.

Causes

The germs involved in vaginal discharge are :

- *Candida albicans, Trichomonas vaginalis, Gardnerella vaginalis*. These germs cause vaginitis.
- *Neisseria gonorrhoeae, Chlamydia trachomatis Mycoplasma genitalium Mycoplasma hominis*. These germs cause cervicitis.

Treatment

- In the case of cervicitis, both gonococcus and chlamydia must be treated.
- Treatment for vaginitis targets *Trichomonas vaginalis, Gardnerella vaginalis and Candida albicans.*

Figure 33: Vaginal discharge algorithm

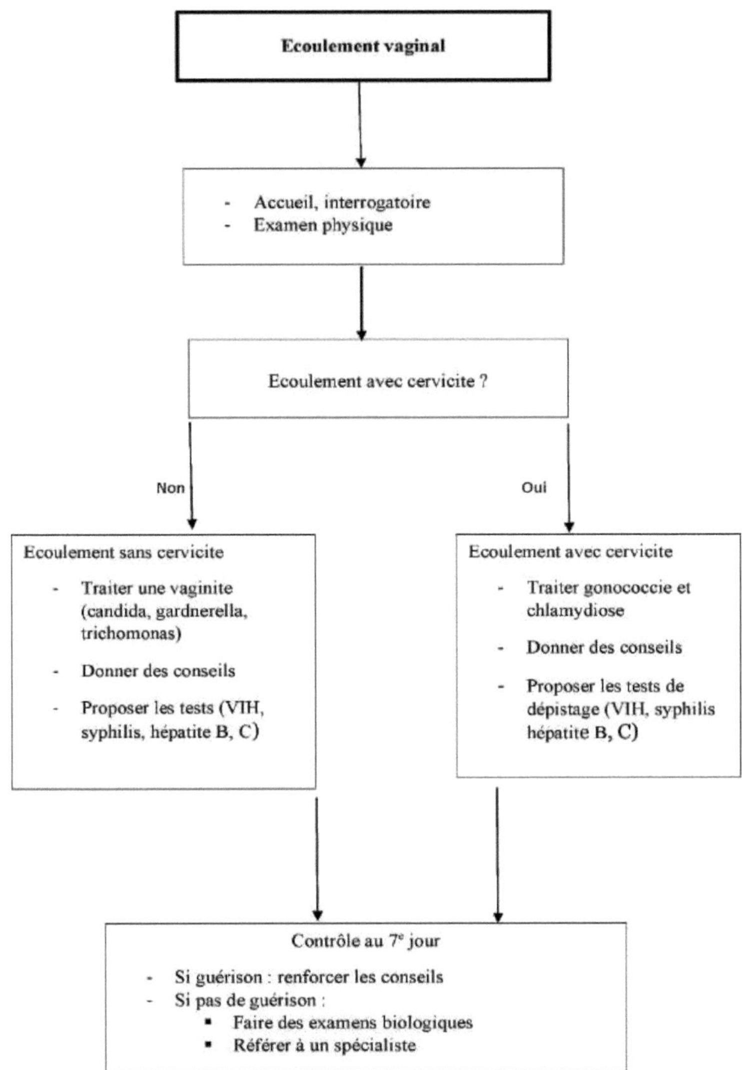

Lower abdominal pain

Lower abdominal pain or pelvic pain, also known as pelvic inflammatory disease or pelvic inflammatory syndrome (PIS), can be caused by an infection of the female pelvic genitalia.

SIP is most often a complication of cervicitis caused by ascending infection with N. *gonorrhoeae* and/or C. *trachomatis* or mycoplasma; sometimes associated with anaerobic germs.

Clinical characteristics

Pelvic pain can be a sign of endometritis, salpingitis, ovaritis or pelviperitonitis, all of which can lead to sterility, extra-uterine pregnancy or death. Therefore, in the event of lower abdominal pain, it is important to look for signs suggestive of an abdominal surgical emergency:

- vaginal bleeding, absence or delay of menstrual periods (extrauterine pregnancy);
- a history of abortion or recent childbirth in the last six weeks;

- tenseness or contracture of the abdominal wall;
- signs of internal bleeding: warmth, thready pulse, low blood pressure;
- signs of appendicitis: pain in the right iliac fossa with fever.

If any of these signs are present, an emergency referral to surgery is required.

In the absence of surgical presentation, if the patient presents with pain provoked by the gynaecological examination, she should be treated for Pelvic Inflammatory Syndrome (PIS).

Causes

Lower abdominal pain can be caused by STI germs (gonococcus, chlamydia, mycoplasma) and/or common germs (anaerobia).

Treatment

In the case of lower abdominal pain, as soon as the surgical emergency has been ruled out, gonococcus, chlamydia, chlamydial infection and other infectious diseases must be treated simultaneously.

Figure 34: Algorithm for lower abdominal pain in women

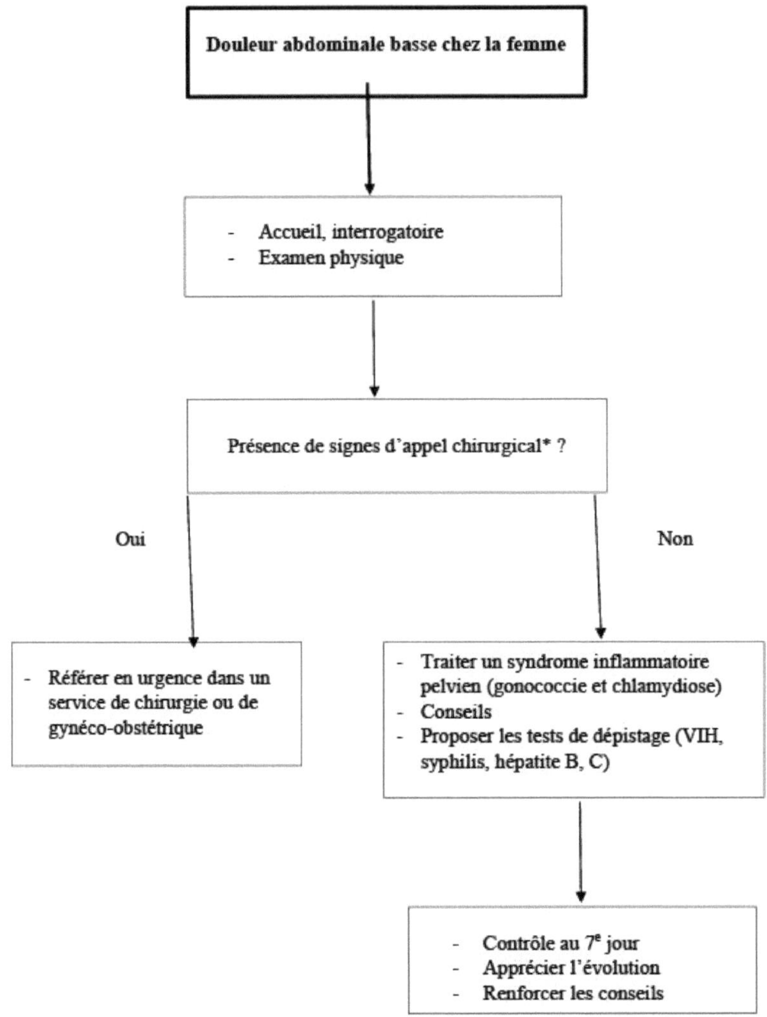

Lower abdominal pain in women

Reception, questioning Physical examination

Presence of surgical warning signs*?

Emergency referral to a surgical or gynaecological obstetrics department

Treating pelvic inflammatory disease (gonorrhoea and chlamydia)

Advice

Offer screening tests (HIV, syphilis, hepatitis B and C)

Day 7 check

Assessing progress

Strengthening advice

* Surgical signs

- Metrorrhagia
- Abdominal defence
- Sign of intestinal obstruction
- Notion of abortion

Tumour of the scrotum

A scrotal tumefaction is an enlargement of the bursa and/or testicles. It may or may not be accompanied by pain.

Clinical characteristics

There may be little or no pain from enlargement of the bursae, or pain in one or both testicles on palpation.

Causes

- *Neisseria gonorrhoeae* (gonorrhoea)
- *Chlamydia trachomatis* (chlamydiosis)

In the event of sudden onset of testicular pain with or without any notion of trauma (testicular torsion); with signs of another surgical pathology, the patient should be referred to a surgical department.

Treatment

Patients with scrotal tumours should be treated simultaneously for gonococcal and chlamydial infections.

Figure 35: Scrotal tumour algorithm

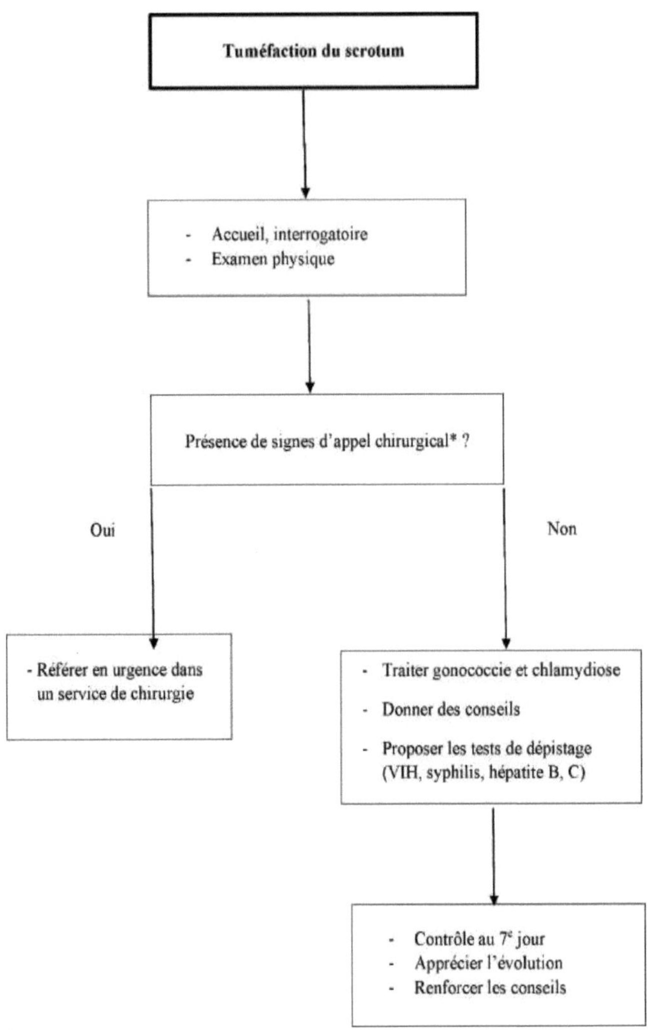

* Surgical signs
- Testicular torsion
- Severe trauma to the scrotum

Genital ulceration

Genital ulceration is a non-traumatic loss of tissue in the skin or mucous membranes of the genitals.

Clinical characteristics. On examination, it may be a :

- single, painless, clean ulceration (syphilis) ;
- ulcerations that are often multiple, deep-rooted, dirty and very painful (chancre mou);
- very superficial ulcerations, grouped together, not very painful, with the notion of vesicles and recurrences (genital herpes);
- small, rarely visible ulceration with little pain (lymphogranulomatosis venereum).

Causes

The most common causes of genital ulceration are as follows:

- *Treponema pallidum* (syphilis)
- *Haemophilus ducreyi* (chancre mou)
- *Chlamydia trachomatis* (lymphogranulomatosis venereum).
- *Herpes simplex virus* (genital herpes)

These different causes may be combined.

Treatment

- Patients suffering from genital ulcers should be treated at the same time for syphilis and chancroid (depending on the epidemiological context, particularly in Africa).

-If vesicles or ulcers recur, genital herpes and syphilis must be treated.

Given the dangers of syphilis for the foetus, treatment of syphilis in pregnant women should be a routine part of any consultation for genital ulceration.

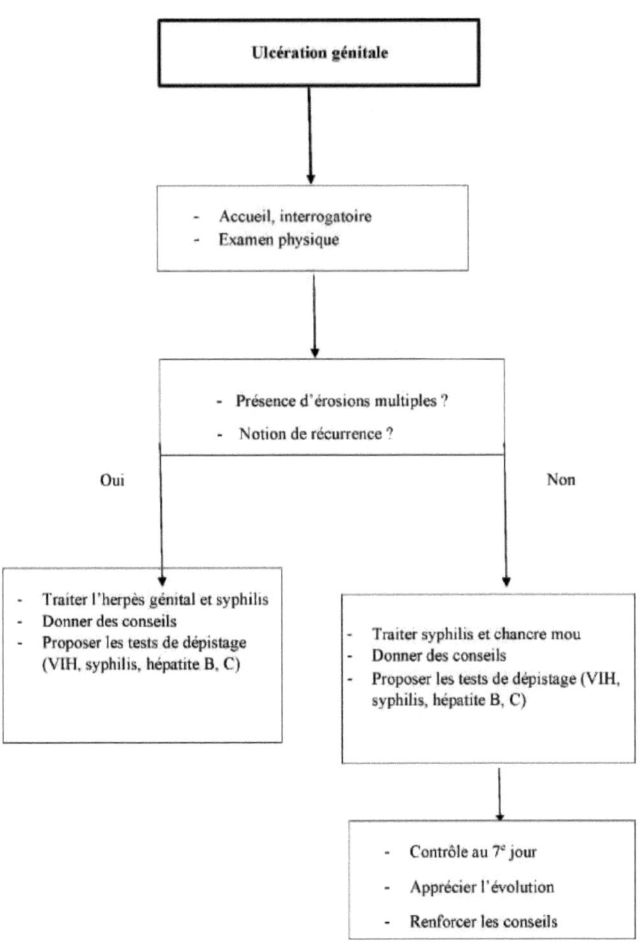
Ulcération génitale
- Accueil, interrogatoire
- Examen physique
- Présence d'érosions multiples ?
- Notion de récurrence ?
Oui
Non
- Traiter l'herpès génital et syphilis
- Donner des conseils
- Proposer les tests de dépistage (VIH, syphilis, hépatite B, C)
- Traiter syphilis et chancre mou
- Donner des conseils
- Proposer les tests de dépistage (VIH, syphilis, hépatite B, C)
- Contrôle au 7e jour
- Apprécier l'évolution
- Renforcer les conseils

Inguinal bubo

The inguinal bubo is a painful or painless, often fluctuating, tumour of the inguinal lymph nodes.

Clinical characteristics

Clinical examination reveals one or more adenopathies, which may or may not be painful, uni or bi-lateral, and may or may not be associated with genital ulceration.

Causes

Chlamydia trachomatis (lymphogranulomatosis venereum).

Haemophilus ducreyi (chancre mou)

Treatment

- Patients presenting with a bubo without genital ulceration should be treated simultaneously for venereal lymphogranulomatosis and chancre mou (depending on the epidemiological context).
- For patients presenting with a bubo with genital ulceration, use the genital ulceration algorithm.

Figure 37: Inguinal bubo algorithm

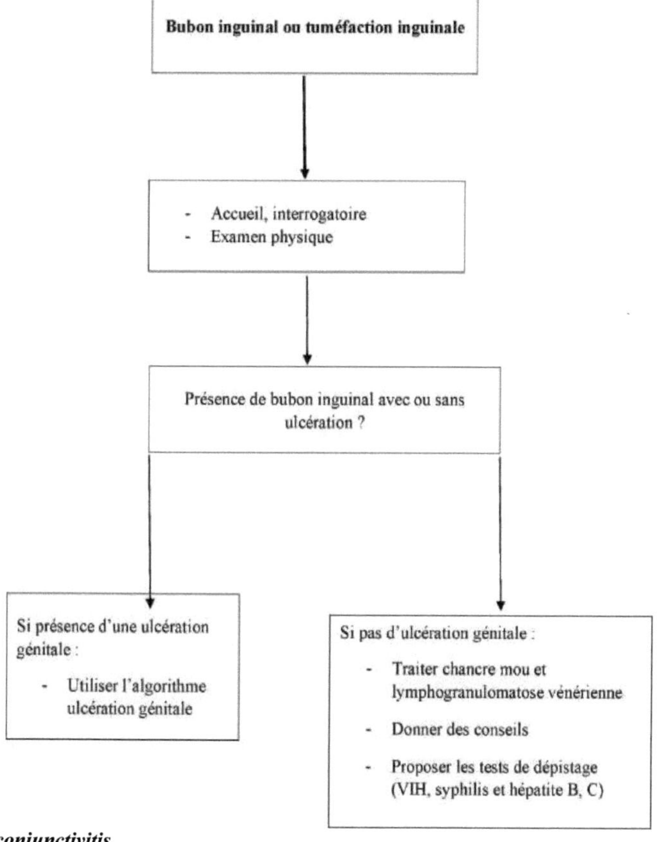

Neonatal conjunctivitis

Neonatal conjunctivitis is a purulent secretion from the eyes. It is an infection contracted in the first month of life during passage through the mother's infected birth canal. Untreated or inadequately treated, this infection can lead to loss of sight in the child (cecitis).

Clinical characteristics

These are :

- purulent secretion from one or both eyes, whether or not associated with redness and/or swelling of the eyelids;
- a simple persistent redness of the eyes.

Causes

- *Neisseria gonorrhoeae* (gonorrhoea)
- *Chlamydia trachomatis* (chlamydiosis)

Treatment

In the case of conjunctivitis in newborns, gonococcal and chlamydial infections in newborns should be treated at the same time, and the mother should also be treated.

Figure 38: Newborn conjunctivitis algorithm

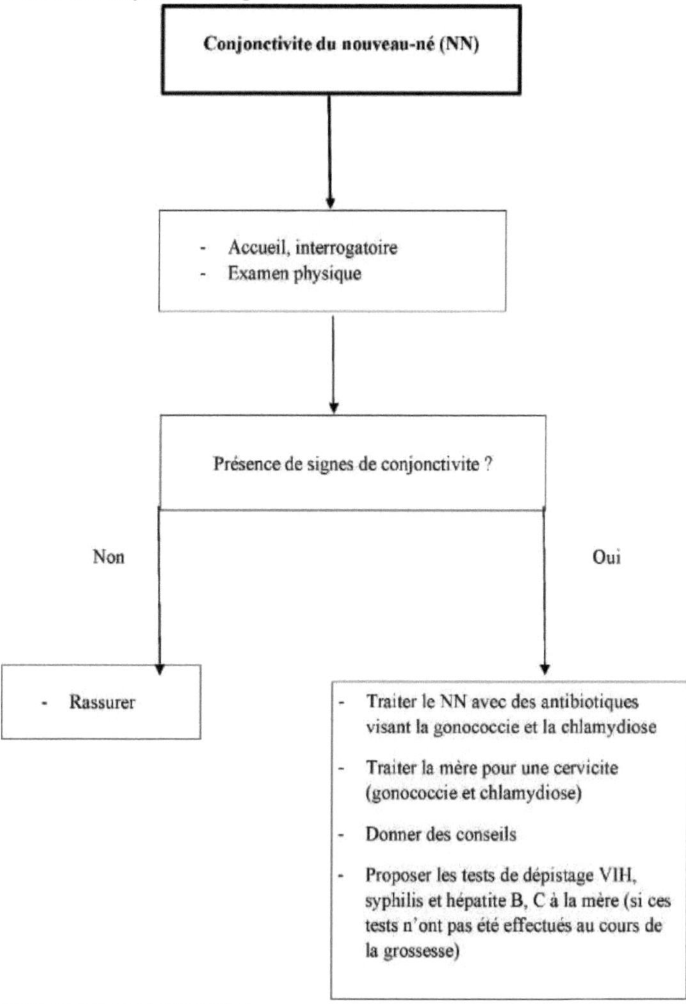

Condylomata or venereal vegetation

Condylomata or venereal vegetations (cocksuckers) are a 1ST tumour of viral origin, contagious and self-inoculating.

Clinical characteristics

Venereal vegetations appear as excrescences, often painless, of variable size, with irregular, sometimes pedunculated surfaces. In men, these lesions may occur on the penis, scrotum, pubis, inguinal folds, urethral meat and anal margin. In women, the lesions occur on the vulva, lips, pubis, inguinal folds, anal margin, vagina and cervix.

Causes

The pathogenic agent is the Human Papilloma Virus (HPV). There are several types. Most of these viruses are responsible for benign anogenital condyloma. Other types of virus are responsible for cervical cancer and can cause cancer of the vulva and penis. When we know that papilloma viruses play an important role in the genesis of cervical cancer, prevention messages, correct treatment and surveillance of young people with condylomas are important in the management of condylomas in both men and women.

Treatment

Condylomata of the cervix and vagina must be treated in a specialised department or any other department equipped with trained staff and appropriate means of treatment.
Condylomata of the external genitalia are treated with liquid nitrogen (cryotherapy), electrocautery (surgical method) or podophyllin diluted to 10 or 25%, depending on the case.

References

1. World Health Organisation. Global program on AIDS. Management of sexually transmitted diseases. WHO Geneva. GPA/TEM/94.1, 1994
2. Grosskurth H, Mosha F, Todd J et al. Impact of improved treatment of sexually transmitted diseases on HIV in rural Tanzania. Randomised controlled trial. Lancet 1995;346;530-6
3. Kapiga SH, Vulstere B, Lyamya EF. Evaluation of sexually transmistted diseases diagnotic among famlily planning clients in Dar es Salam Tanzanya. Sex Transm Infect 1998; 74(Suppl1) :S132-8
4. Programme national de lutte contre le Sida et les IST (Togo Ministry of Health). Guide national de prise en charge des IST, Edition 2017, Lome
5. Moges B, Yismaw G, Kassu A, et al. Sexually transmitted infections based on the syndromic approach in Gondar town, northwest Ethiopia: a retrospective study.. BMC Public Health. 2013;13:143.
6. Redwood-Campbell L, Plumb J.J The syndromic approach to treatment of sexually transmitted diseases in low-income countries: issues, challenges, and future directions. Obstet Gynaecol Can 2002; 24:417-24.
7. La Ruche G, Djeha D, Boka-Yao A et al. The fight against sexually transmitted diseases in Ivory Coast: what strategies can we use in the face of HIV/AIDS? Sante 2000;10:287-92.
8. La Ruche G, Lorougnon F, Digbeu N. Therapeutic algorithms for the management of sexually transmitted diseases at the peripheral level in Cote d'Ivoire: assessment of efficacy and cost. Bull World Health Organ 1995;73:305-13.
9. Alary M, Baganizi E, Guedeme A et al. Evaluation of clinical algorithm for the diagnosis of gonococcal and chlamydial infection among men with urethral discharge or dysuria and women with vaginal discharge in Benin. Sex Transm Infect 1998; 17 (Suppl1) : S44-9
10. Bitere R, Alary M, Viens P et al. Qualite de la prise en charge des maladies sexuellement transmissibles en Afrique de l'Ouest ; enquete aupres de six pays. Cahiers Sante 2002; 12; 233-9
12. Ferreira A, Young T, Mathews C et al. Strategies for partner notification for sexually transmitted infections, including HIV. Cochrane Database Syst Rev 2013;2013(10):CD002843. doi: 10.1002/14651858.CD002843.
13. Gupta V, Sharma VK. Syndromic management of sexually transmitted infections: A critical appraisal and the road ahead. Natl Med J India 2019;32:147-152
14. Wi TE, Ndowa FJ, Ferreyra C et al. Diagnosing sexually transmitted infections in resource-constrained settings: challenges and ways forward.
J Int AIDS Soc 2019; Suppl 6:e25343. doi: 10.1002/jia2.2534
15. World Health Organization. Guidelines for the management of symptomatic sexually transmitted infections. Geneva: World Health Organization; 2021.
16. Almugti HS, Al Hakeem RN, Alghamdi AM et al. Assessment of using the syndromic approach in managing patients with sexually transmitted diseases among the national guard primary health care physicians, Jeddah City, Saudi Arabia.
Cureus 2022;14:e21502. doi: 10.7759/cureus.21502. eCollection 2022
17. Vuylsteke B. Current status of syndromic management of sexually transmitted infections in developing countries. Sex Transm Infect 2004;80:333-4
18. Moherdaui F, Vuylsteke B, Siqueira LF et al. Validation of national algorithms for the

diagnosis of sexually transmitted diseases in Brazil: results from a multicentre study. Sex Transm Infect 1998;74 (Suppl) 1:S38-43.
19. Vuylsteke BL, Ettiegne-Traore V, Anoma CK et al. Assessment of the validity of and adherence to sexually transmitted infection algorithms at a female sex worker clinic in Abidjan, Cote d'Ivoire. Sex Transm Dis 2003;30 :284-91
20. De Baetselier I, Vuylsteke B, Yaya I et al. To pool or not to pool samples for sexually transmitted infections detection in MSM ? An evaluation of a new pooling method using the GeneXpert Instrument in West Africa. Sex Transm Dis 2020; 47:556-561.
21. Lutz AR. Screening for asymptomatic extragenital gonorrhea and chlamydia in MSM. Significance, recommendations, and options for overcoming barriers to testing. LGBT Health. 2015; 2:27-34.

PART X

X. Management of a programme to combat STIs

1. Development process and content of a programme or project 1ST

As with any public health programme, the first step is to carry out an analysis of the epidemiological situation (determining the prevalence and causes of 1ST, identifying the most vulnerable populations) and the programmatic situation (determining the services offered or existing, identifying the areas of coverage, identifying the gaps in terms of services to be covered, and the needs for capacity building in terms of technical and human resources) [1-4]. The data obtained from the situation analysis will be used to draw up a strategic plan and/or a results-based action (or operational) plan.

The action plan must be complete and contain key elements:

- objectives, strategies and actions to be undertaken and their timetable ;
- priority target populations ;
- the package of services to be offered ;
- the programme coverage area ;
- duration or period of the plan ;
- Estimated budget for activities and resource mobilisation strategy ;
- measurable indicators (process and impact indicators) ;
- the stakeholders involved in implementation.

To implement the programme smoothly and effectively, we need :

- agree on its components with all stakeholders,
- draw up standards and procedures for implementing the components,
- draw up management guidelines with algorithms and therapeutic protocols based on scientific evidence (germs and levels of antibiotic resistance),
- agree on effective input management mechanisms (stock supply management: SSM)
- draw up and implement a training programme for health professionals and community workers in the field, who will be involved at all levels of implementation,
- set up an effective programme monitoring and evaluation system.

2. Main components of an IST programme or project [5-7]

- Prevention (primary and secondary)
- Effective diagnosis and treatment of cases
- Training
- Monitoring and evaluation
- Operational research

3. Standards and procedures

For the smooth and effective implementation of a 1ST management programme in the field (at the level of a country or geographical area covered by the programme), a document defining the standards and procedures is required. In practice, if standards and procedures already exist in the country, they should be adopted, revised or adapted as necessary. If not, however, these standards must be drawn up and validated by all the stakeholders involved in implementing the project or programme. Depending on the case, the experience of national institutions (ministry responsible for health, or public health programmes) or international institutions and non-governmental organisations in drawing up standards and procedures documents may be used [8-11].

These standards and procedures should be developed and disseminated to all stakeholders in the programme or project. The aim of standards and procedures is quality assurance of care and services [8, 9, 11]. Quality assurance encompasses the technical standards of care providers and managers on the one hand, and the quality lost by the patient on the other.

The norms or standards define for each component :

- the minimum package of services to be offered at each level of the health pyramid;

- beneficiaries of services ;
- service providers according to their qualifications and skills ;
- minimum equipment ;
- the times and frequency at which services must be provided ;

The standards specify the minimum acceptable level of performance for each activity.

The *procedures* describe, in a chronological and precise manner, the actions involved in carrying out a task in order to achieve a minimum acceptable level of service delivery. Protocols are linked to IST service standards.

In a health programme, standards and procedures are applied to all components.

3.1. Prevention

STI prevention is the set of interventions that enable patients or the general public to adopt behaviours that reduce the risk of STI/HIV transmission.

The objectives of STI prevention are to :

- reduce the incidence and prevalence of STIs in the population ;
- promote behaviour that reduces the risk of STI transmission;
- promote access to healthcare, particularly for the most vulnerable groups;

Prevention initiatives focus on **:**

- behaviour change communication (BCC) ;
- the use of condoms ;
- promoting the use of healthcare services.

3.1.1 Standards

- The talk

The 1ST talk is a planned group discussion, facilitated by service providers, to get members of a group to analyse a specific problem and to help them adopt health-promoting behaviour. To ensure that everyone can take part, the number of participants in the talk should not exceed 20.

Service providers :

- formal health agents ;
- trained peer educators ;
- opinion leader ;
- association members ;
- communicators ;
- community relays ;
- social agents.

Time

The talk can be :

- while customers wait for their consultation;
- as part of advanced strategies ;
- by appointment for specific groups.

Levels

- Peripheral,
- Intermediary.
- Central.

Equipment

- Audiovisual equipment: sound films; television set; video recorder, videos (CD, DVD USB); megaphone;
- Visual and graphic materials: posters; billboards; photos; image boxes; leaflets; demonstration materials (mannequins, condoms).

Location: consultation room; waiting room; counselling room

The venue must be easy to get to, comfortable, sufficiently spacious, well lit and airy.

Target groups / Beneficiaries

- General population,
- Vulnerable groups.
- Counselling / Interpersonal Communication (IPC)

Counselling/CIP is a dialogue between a provider and a patient, with the aim of making the patient aware of his or her risk behaviour, identifying his or her problems, expressing them and considering possible solutions for changing behaviour.

Providers: *trained health workers; trained community health workers.*

Levels (at all levels of the health pyramid)

- Peripheral; intermediate; central.

Equipment :

- demonstration media ;
- condoms (M/F).

Location

- consultation room ;
- examination room ;
- boardroom.

Target groups / Beneficiaries

- STI patients ;
- sexual partners.
- Raising awareness through the mass media

The mass media are defined as all the communication channels used to reach a target audience. These different channels are :

- *Written press*: advertising pages and slogans; articles.
- *Radio:* advertising spots and slogans; radio messages on STIs; sketches on STIs; radio debates; interactive programmes.
- *Television: commercials*, slogans, televised messages; songs, theatre and sketches; televised debates.
- *Social networks:* website, Facebook, YouTube, Instagram, tiktok, etc.

Service providers

- health agents ;
- opinion leader ;
- members of associations and NGOs ;
- communicators ;
- peer educators ;
- social agents.

Levels: peripheral; intermediate; central.

Target/beneficiary groups: general population.

3.1.2 Procedures

- Organising a group chat

The subject. You need :

- Gather as much information as possible about the group you are going to meet;
- choose a presentation topic of interest to the whole group;
- make sure the subject is simple ;
- prepare a short list of the most important points;
- focus on the behaviours we would like participants to adopt with regard to STDs and HIV/AIDS.

The knowledge, attitudes or practices that you want people to acquire are the objectives of your presentation.

Methods

- The method must be participatory;
- If you are presenting information, posters can be useful;
- If we are teaching new skills, a demonstration would be necessary;

- If you want the group to reflect on their attitudes and values, stories and proverbs can help.

Preparation:

- make an outline of the presentation ;
- try to repeat the whole presentation;
- check that all the equipment is useful and corresponds to what is expected;
- ask someone to observe one of your "repetitions";
- make the necessary corrections before meeting your audience;
- ensure that the presentation does not exceed 30 minutes, including discussion and questions;
- The timing is crucial: choose a time when there are enough patients or participants and when they are most attentive;

The venue for the presentation must be chosen after determining what is most convenient for customers;

- preparation includes gathering all the material in advance so that it is ready to hand when the presentation begins;
- ensure that the language of communication is appropriate for the audience.

Putting it into practice

People will learn more from a presentation if they are asked to participate actively:

- After explaining what you want to talk about, always ask your audience to tell you what they already know about the subject;
- encourage participation, whatever the method used.

When you show a poster, immediately ask what they think. After telling a story, ask questions to find out everyone's opinions.

Whenever a technique is demonstrated, care must be taken to ensure that each participant can practise the task in question.

Evaluation: at the end of the talk, check what the audience has retained.

Conclusion: say thank you and arrange the next appointment.

- Organisation of counselling /CIP

Preparation. You will need :

- ensuring confidentiality ;
- make sure the room is well ventilated and lit;
- make sure that tables and chairs are available;
- Gather visual aids (posters, diagrams, leaflets) ;
- ensure that documentation is available (patient files, daily activity register, monitoring form).

The stages of interpersonal communication about STIs

Good interpersonal communication involves a number of important steps, from the conditions in which patients are received and examined to information about the disease and the behaviour to adopt.

► Exam interview conditions

- Conditions must be in place to ensure confidentiality (interview room and conditions);
- Reassure the patient about the confidentiality of the interview (the information exchanged between the provider and the patient is confidential and must not be communicated to a third party without the patient's authorisation.

► Specific information

They include information about the infection and how to treat it.

<u>Information on the disease :</u>

- Inform patients about their STI;
- Explain how it was transmitted and how to prevent it from spreading;
- Describe complications if they are not treated;
- Describe other STI symptoms and ask the patient to come back if they notice any symptoms.

<u>Information on treatment :</u>

- Explain the treatment to the patient and how to reduce symptoms if the disease is viral;

- Explain to the patient that they should abstain from sexual intercourse until the treatment has been completed, or that they should use condoms;
- If necessary, show the patient how to use the condom.
- Requires a follow-up appointment.
- Remind the patient of the importance of a follow-up appointment after treatment
- Assure patients that they can return to the same clinic if they need advice and medical care.

► Taking care of partners
- Explain to the patient that his partner must be well treated;
- Ask how you can help him to bring his partners for treatment or give the patient the prescription for his partners;
- Ensuring confidentiality, availability and quality of service for its partners.
- HIV risk assessment and personal risk reduction plan
- Inform patients that they are at risk of HIV infection;
- Discuss the possible consequences of high-risk behaviour (sexual behaviour, use of alcohol, tobacco and other drugs);
- Explain safe sex practices and how condoms can reduce the risk of STI/HIV transmission;
- Inform them about HIV testing;

► Double protection
- Explain the principle of dual protection to the patient and encourage him or her to choose one of the two options.

appropriate method.
- For young people, explain the advantages of using condoms to avoid STIs/HIV and unwanted pregnancies (double protection).

► Offer HIV, syphilis and viral hepatitis B and C screening tests

It is important to offer all STI patients (who are already at risk) screening for other STIs to ensure early, holistic treatment.

3.2 Early and effective management of 1ST

Early and effective management of 1ST consists of diagnosing and treating any patient complaining of STI symptoms at the first consultation, in accordance with national guidelines.
The objectives of early and effective care are to :
- prevent the development of disease, complications and sequelae ;
- interrupting the chain of transmission of infections contracted during sexual relations ;
- reduce the risk of HIV infection.

Early and effective care is based on three main activities:
- case management at the first consultation ;
- management of referrals ;
- management of asymptomatic cases.

3.2.1 Standards
- Case management at the first consultation

The management of STI cases during the first consultation is based on the syndromic or etiological approach, depending on the country and the availability of suitable technical facilities.
Service providers
Health workers trained in this syndromic approach, in particular doctors and paramedics (nurses and midwives, or health technicians).
Premises and equipment:
- suitable, well-lit, well-ventilated premises, ensuring confidentiality;
- data collection media ;
- treatment algorithms ;
- minimum equipment required.

Target groups / beneficiaries :

- symptomatic STI patients ;
- sexual partners.
- Management of referrals

This is the management of cases referred by the establishment for initial consultation, or presenting a proven failure to respond to first-line treatment, or patients with non-curable STIs (such as condyloma or herpetic recurrence, or pelvic inflammatory syndromes in women). The aim is to ensure that patients receive the most appropriate and qualified care. The treatment of STI referrals is based exclusively on an etiological approach.

Service providers :
- biologists ;
- general practitioners with a laboratory ;
- specialist doctors.

Premises and equipment
- The clinical premises and equipment must meet the same standards as for the initial consultation.
- Biological premises and equipment must meet laboratory standards for etiological diagnosis
- Data collection media.

Target groups / beneficiaries :
- patient referrals ;
- patients who have failed first-line treatment.
- Management of asymptomatic cases

In many cases, STIs have no symptoms at all. These may be curable infections such as gonorrhoea, chlamydia and syphilis, or non-curable infections, usually viral, such as genital herpes and papilloma virus.

Two strategies are known to be effective in detecting and managing these cases. These are :
- screening for syphilis and viral hepatitis in pregnant women and certain high-risk groups such as sex workers and men who have sex with men;
- notification of partners (management of partners using the same treatment regimens as syndromic cases).

Screening for syphilis in pregnant women and at-risk groups *(sex workers, men who have sex with men)*

Service providers :
- Any authorised provider or provider of prenatal consultations;
- Biologist and laboratory technician.

Premises and equipment :
- Laboratory team ;
- Suitable clinical premises and equipment;
- Syphilis screening kits and accessories,
- Data collection media.

Target groups ;
Pregnant women;
Sex workers ;
Men who have sex with other men.

Notification of partners

The aim is to take all the necessary steps (providing informed information to the patient) in collaboration with the patient consulting for an STI to ensure that his or her sexual partner is taken care of, in order to break the chain of transmission and avoid any complications. *Providers:* any provider trained in the management of 1ST.

Material:
- Notification form ;

- Invitation to tender.
- Telephone (SMS messages, WhatsApp, calls, etc.)

Target groups/beneficiaries

Partner in any case :

- of urethral flow ;
- genital ulcers :
- of venereal vegetation.

Table 17: Standards for the early and effective management of 1ST

ACTIVITIES	SERVICE SUPPLIERS			PREMISES AND EQUIPMENT	j TARGET GROUPS ' / BENEFICIARIES
	Nurses Midwives	*General practitioners*	*Specialist doctors Biologists*		
1. Case management at the first consultation	+	+	+	- Local adapts : - Management algorithms - Minimum equipment (list attached)	- Symptomatic 1ST patients - Their sexual partners.
2. Management of referrals	-	+	+	Adapted premises and laboratories for each level (see attached list)	- Reference cases - Previous treatment failures
3. Management of asymptomatic cases 3.1. Screening for syphilis in pregnant women	+	+	+	- Syphilis screening kits and accessories - Data collection support - Suitable premises	-Pregnant women
pregnant women and certain at-risk groups 3.2. Notification of partners	+	+	+	- Notification forms - Invitation to consultation	- Partners in lST cases

3.2.2 Procedures

- Case management at the first consultation

This care consists of :

- ensuring a warm welcome (establishing a climate of trust and confidentiality) ;
- carry out a correct clinical examination: questioning; examination of the external genitalia; general examination;
- make a diagnosis;
- prescribe appropriate treatment in accordance with national guidelines (algorithms) ;
- give appropriate advice;
- promoting the use of condoms;
- offer screening tests (HIV, syphilis, hepatitis B and C);
- make a follow-up appointment;
- register and notify cases.
- Management of referrals

It follows the same steps as the initial consultation. However, diagnosis and treatment are based on the etiological approach. In addition, feedback must be provided to the referring provider.

3.3. TRAINING

Training in the management of 1ST is a process designed to impart the knowledge and skills required for the effective management of STIs. Its aim is to enhance providers' knowledge and skills in the prevention and management of STIs.

3.3.1 Standards

The types of training required are Clinical training ;

Biological training ;
Supervision training ;
Training in monitoring/evaluation ;

- Clinical training

The aim is to improve the knowledge, skills and attitudes of providers in the management of STIs.
Service providers (trainers)
- STI specialists
- Formed general practitioners

Equipment
- Adapted premises ;
- Trainer's guide
- National reference documents and manuals (national STI management guide, national document on standards and procedures)
- Workbook ;
- Teaching materials.

Beneficiaries
- Public and private IST service providers at all levels;
- Programme managers ;
- Supervisors.
- Biology training

The aim is to strengthen skills in the screening and etiological diagnosis of 1ST.
Service providers (trainers) :
- central and intermediate level biologists ;
- university teachers ;
- biological engineers ;

Premises and equipment:
- suitable premises ;
- trainer's guide ;
- national reference documents and manuals (national STI management guide, national document on standards and procedures, etc.);
- internship notebook ;
- teaching materials ;
- laboratory equipment and products.

Target groups / beneficiaries :
- laboratory technicians ;
- medical biologists :
- pharmacist-biologists.
- Supervision training

Supervision training consists of developing providers' skills so that they are able to use the facilitating approach of supervising service providers on their work site to improve the health facility's performance.
Providers (trainers): qualified resource persons
Premises and equipment:
- suitable premises ;
- trainer's guide ;
- national reference documents and manuals (national STI management guide, national document on standards and procedures, etc.);
- course notebooks.

Target groups / beneficiaries :
- programme managers ;

- clinicians working in facilities offering STI services;
- pharmacy managers ;
- laboratory managers.
- Training in monitoring and evaluation

Training in monitoring/evaluation consists of strengthening the skills of service providers in :
- deciding which activities to monitor and evaluate ;
- planning monitoring and evaluation ;
- monitoring programme activities ;
- evaluate the programme (impact and effect indicators).

Service providers (trainers) :
- consultants (national and international monitoring/evaluation experts),
- programme managers ;
- supervisors;
- doctors;
- pharmacy managers;
- laboratory managers.

Premises and equipment:
- suitable premises;
- trainer's guide;
- national reference documents and manuals (national STI management guide, national document on standards and procedures, etc.);
- internship notebook;
- teaching materials.

Target groups / beneficiaries :
- programme managers ;
- social workers ;
- STI service providers :
- members of NGOs/Associations :
- laboratory technicians.
- Training in Behaviour Change Communication (BCC)

This is the set of activities that contribute to strengthening the skills of CCC service providers.

Providers (trainers): resource persons.

Premises and equipment:
- suitable premises;
- trainer's guide;
- national reference documents and manuals (national STI management guide, national document on standards and procedures, etc.);
- internship notebook;
- teaching materials.

Target groups / beneficiaries :
- health agents;
- social workers;
- community agents;
- opinion leaders;
- communicators;
- peer educators;
- members of associations and NGOs.
- *Infection prevention training*

This refers to all activities aimed at strengthening the skills of service providers in order to prevent infections.

Providers (trainers): resource persons.
Premises and equipment:
- suitable premises ;
- trainer's guide ;
- national reference documents and manuals (national STI management guide, national document on standards and procedures, etc.);
- internship notebook ;
- teaching materials.

Target groups / beneficiaries ;
- health agents ;
- support staff.
- Management training

This is the set of activities that enable providers to have skills in managing medical inputs (medicines, consumables, laboratory products, condoms and other reproductive health products).
Service providers (trainers) :
- resource persons (experts) ;
- programme managers ;
- supervisors ;
- doctors;
- pharmacy managers ;
- laboratory managers.

Premises and equipment:
- suitable premises ;
- national reference documents and manuals (national STI management guide, national document on standards and procedures, etc.);
- trainer's guide ;
- internship notebook ;
- teaching materials.

Target groups / beneficiaries :
- programme managers ;
- social workers ;
- STI service providers ;
- NGO/Association members ;
- laboratory technicians ;
- agents for pharmacies and pharmaceutical depots ;
- point of sale agents.

Table 18: Training standards

ACTIVITIES	PREMISES AND EQUIPMENT			TARGET GROUPS/ BENEFICIARIES
	University teaching consultants	Programme managers, Central staff		

1. CLINICAL TRAINING	+	+	- Adapted premises -Trainer's guide - National reference documents - Work placement notebook - Teaching	- Public and private 1ST service providers at all levels - Programme managers - Supervisors
2. TRAINING IN BIOLOGY	+	+	- Adapted premises - Trainer's guide - National reference documents - Work placement notebook - Teaching materials - Laboratory equipment and	- Laboratory technicians - Medical biologists - Pharmacist biologists
3. SUPERVISION TRAINING	+	+	- Adapted premises - Trainer's guide - National reference documents - Work placement notebook -Teaching materials	- Programme managers - Clinicians working in facilities offering 1ST services - Regional and health district staff - Pharmacy managers - Laboratory managers
TRAINING IN MONITORING/EVALUATION N	+	+	- Adapted premises - Trainer's guide - National reference documents - Work placement notebook - Teaching materials	- Programme managers - Social workers - Service providers 1ST - NGO/Association members - Laboratory technicians
5. TRAINING IN CCC	+	+	- Adapted premises - Trainer's guide -National reference documents - Work placement notebook - Teaching materials	- Health agents - Social workers - Community agents - Opinion leaders - Communicators - Peer educators
6. INFECTION PREVENTION TRAINING	+	+	- Adapted premises - Trainer's guide - National reference documents	- Health agents - Support staff

			- Work placement notebook - Teaching materials	
7. TRAINING MANAGEMENT	+	+	- Adapted premises - Trainer's guide - National reference documents - Work placement notebook - Teaching materials	- Programme managers -Social workers - Service providers 1ST -Members of NGOs/Associations -Laboratory technicians - Agents for pharmacies and pharmaceutical depots - Point of sale agents

3.2.2. Procedures

- **Preparatory activities for the course**
- Assessing training needs ;
- Defining training objectives ;
- Choosing training methods and techniques ;
- Identify the people to be trained ;

92

- Identify facilitators and trainers ;
- Determining the resources required ;
- Mobilising resources ;
- Drawing up a training calendar ;
- Inform participants and check their availability;
- Choose your training venue ;
- Hold a meeting with the facilitators and trainers;
- Pre- and post-test preparation.
- **Training process**
- Welcoming participants;
- Defining work standards ;
- Gather participants' expectations of the course;
- Inform participants about the administrative provisions ;
- Administer the course in accordance with the reference documents;
- Evaluating training.
- **Post-training activities**
- Writing a training report ;
- Distribute the training report ;
- Drawing up and implementing a training follow-up plan.

3.4. Supervision

Supervision is a process which consists of gathering information on the performance, motivation and working conditions of the staff member being supervised, with a view to improving the quality of service delivery. Its objectives are to guide, support and assist staff to enable them to carry out their assigned tasks effectively.

3.4.1 Standards

The areas to be supervised in the fight against 1ST are :

- behaviour change communication (BCC) ;

- Treatment of STIs ;
- management of medicines, condoms and laboratory products ;
- Working conditions.

Service providers (supervisors) :
- programme managers ;
- chief district medical officer ;
- form supervisors
- formal health agents
- social agents forms

The supervisor must be a model of competence and performance.

Material:
- supervision grid ;
- job description ;
- standards and procedures ;
- supervision guide.

Target groups (supervisors) :
- healthcare workers (healthcare providers, laboratory technicians, medical input managers) ;
- social workers and community workers

Table 19: Supervision standards

AREAS	SERVICE SUPPLIERS	MATERIAL	TARGET SUPERVISES
	Health officer and programme resource person		
CCC *	+	Supervision grid/ Job description N P** document	Health workers Social workers Community leaders
Taking charge of SI^r	+	Supervisory grid Job description N P document	Health personnel
Management of medicines, condoms and laboratory products	+	Supervisory grid/ Job description N P document	Pharmacist Pharmacy staff or pharmacist's depot Laboratory technician
Working conditions	+	Supervisory grid Job description N P document	All service providers on the site

3.4.2 Procedures

Preparing for the supervision visit
- Drawing up the supervision schedule;
- Inform the staff to be supervised and negotiate the date;
- Draw up the supervisor's visit plan;
- Defining the objectives of supervision ;
- Determine the activities and tasks to be supervised and carried out;
- Choosing the right monitoring tools ;
- Determining the type of supervision to be carried out;
- Assessing the resources required;

Examine the health facility's documents.

Executing supervision

Meet the head of the health centre and the staff.
- Review the supervision plan and discuss the aims and objectives of the visit;
- Explain how the visit will be conducted;
- Review the recommendations and commitments made during the last monitoring visit;
- Discuss the supervision of different areas of activity;
- Arrange a problem-solving meeting with the training team
- health.

Supervising the various areas of activity.
- Organise a meeting with staff to discuss the strengths and weaknesses of the programme and short- and long-term solutions;
- Organise a summary meeting with the health facility manager;
- Drawing up a problem-solving plan with staff.

Post-supervision activities
- Draw up a supervision report, a copy of which will be sent to the health facility being supervised and another to the supervisor;
- Follow the problem-solving plan.

3.5. Monitoring and evaluation

Monitoring consists of identifying and recording the programme's events, activities, people and material resources. It is based on continuous or periodic data collection. Evaluation involves measuring the extent to which the objectives set have been achieved, and taking corrective action or making decisions for the future of the programme. Monitoring activities helps to evaluate projects and programmes, and to improve the quality and performance of services.

3.5.1 Standards
- Monitoring and evaluation indicators
- National health policy on STIs ;
- The organisation of the healthcare system ;
- National priorities ;
- Unmet needs.

Care provision and *quality*
- Number of consultations ;
- Number of condoms distributed ;
- The number of new cases managed on a syndromic basis.

Staff efficiency
- Number and distribution according to workload ;
- Initial and continuing training.

User satisfaction and response
- Workload due to STIs ;
- Type of patients using STI services ;
- Attendance rates at health centres;
- The proportion of patients who consider the facility to be their first option.

Needs and resource allocation
- Monitoring operating costs;
- Salaries, travel expenses ;
- Supplies, medicines, laboratory products and condoms;
- Initial investment ;
- Types of assessment

The IST programme must undergo at least one initial, one intermediate and one final evaluation. This evaluation may be internal, external or mixed: - The initial or final evaluation must be external or mixed;
- The interim evaluation may be internal or mixed.

Profile of evaluators (Providers): All evaluations will be carried out by qualified individuals with the required skills.
Material : Evaluation documents (protocol validated by stakeholders)
Dissemination of results: The results of any evaluation will be the subject of a written report which will be sent within a reasonable time (no more than three months after the evaluation) to those responsible for the programmes and to all the partners concerned.
Table 20: Monitoring standards

ACTIVITIES	SERVICE SUPPLIERS				AREAS
	Ministry of Health			Development partners Donors and cooperation agencies	
	Programme Manager	*Staff of the epidemiology units*	*Executive bodies*		
Periodic activities	+	+		+	Level of achievement Constraints Use of resources
Coordination meetings	+	+	+	+	Level of implementation of the operational plan Constraints Use of resources Continuation of the operational plan
Monitoring	+	+	+	+	Programme indicators Programme objectives Activities Activity indicators Expected level of achievement Practices and results

Table 21: Valuation standards

ACTIVITIES	SERVICE SUPPLIERS					AREAS
	External assessor	***Ministry of Health***			***Development partner Donors and cooperation agencies***	
		Programme Manager	***Epidemiology unit staff***	***Bodies implementing activities in the field***		
Evaluation Initiate	**+**	**+**	**+**	**+**	**+**	-National priorities -Unmet needs -Existing services -community
Evaluation Intermediate	**+**	**+**	**+**	**+**	**+**	-Level of achievement of results -Constraints -Use of resources
Evaluation Final	**+**	**+**	**+**	**+**	**+**	-Level of achievement of objectives -Constraints -Use of resources -National priorities -Unmet needs

5.5.2. Procedures

▪ ***Follow-up***

Organisation of a coordination meeting

► Preparation

- Determine the order of the day;
- Identify participants ;
- Fix the date, place and time of the meeting;
- Inform participants at least one week before the start of the meeting;
- Gather the necessary documents and teaching aids;
- Decide how decisions are to be made.
- Animation
- Designing a moderator/session chair ;
- Designate a secretary for the meeting ;
- Adopt the agenda;
- Allocate time according to the agenda;
- Ensure that the meeting is focused and progresses smoothly;
- Summarise the decisions taken at the end of each game;
- Conclude the meeting and set the date for the next meeting.
- Post-meeting activities
- Writing the report ;
- Discuss the report with the participants to obtain their additions and corrections;

Organisation of a meeting of field activities

- Organise the list of items to be followed by type of operation
- Programme indicators ;
- Programme objectives ;
- Activities ;
- Activity indicators ;
- Expected level of achievement ;
- Practices and results.

► Select the main elements to be monitored

- Take the following criteria into account;
- Link between the indicator and certain major activities to be carried out during the year ;
- Existence of a method for quantifying the indicator ;
- Link between the indicator and the programme objectives.
- Plan the monitoring of activities
- Choosing monitoring methods ;
- Periodic or systematic reports ;
- Visits and supervision reports ;
- Specifying the frequency of monitoring ;
- The intervals must be sufficiently regular for problems to be identified and resolved in good time.

► Monitoring activities

- Supervise those responsible for each operation;
- Establish a system for supervising all staff adequately.

Use monitoring results to identify problems and propose solutions

- Evaluation

Preparation

- Drawing up terms of reference;
- Defining objectives ;
- Setting up the evaluation team ;

- Identifying the evaluation method and tools ;
- Gathering reference documents;
- Identify the players and sites to visit;
- Setting up a calendar ;
- List the activities to be carried out in the field;
- Communicate the timetable to players and sites;
- Communicating objectives and activities to stakeholders and sites ;
- Assemble equipment if necessary (support and logistics).

Meeting at the start of the evaluation

- Introducing the evaluation team ;
- Present the aims and objectives of the evaluation ;
- Present the activities planned during the evaluation ;
- Identify the people directly involved in the evaluation;
- Discuss the evaluation activities and timetable with the participants.

On-site assessment

Use assessment tools to :

- Observing an STI talk session;
- Observe STI clinical standards and procedures;
- Observe infection prevention standards and procedures;
- Observe working conditions (premises and equipment);
- Observe the management of medicines and condoms;
- Ask customers for their views on the services offered.

Post-evaluation activities

Organise an end-of-assessment meeting to :

- Reintroduce the devaluation team;
- Review the aims and objectives of the evaluation ;
- Present the findings and conclusions of the evaluation;
- Propose recommendations.

Finalising the assessment

- Writing the evaluation report;
- Send the reports to the national authorities and/or development partners who financed the evaluation;
- Disseminate the report to the various stakeholders and partners involved in the programme and/or who took part in the evaluation.

3.6. Epidemiological surveillance of STIs

Epidemiological surveillance of STIs is a continuous and systematic process of collecting, analysing, interpreting and disseminating data on STIs with a view to making decisions and taking action.

3.6.1 Standards

The five components of STI epidemiological surveillance required for an effective programme are as follows: - notification of cases;

- prevalence studies;
- study of the etiology of STI syndromes;
- monitoring antibiotic resistance;
- special studies (socio-behavioural studies, service quality assessment, etc.).

These components are important activities in the effective fight against STIs.

- Syndromic notification

This is a notification process for STIs diagnosed by syndromic approach and recorded during consultations. It involves the management of the sexual partners of patients received and treated in health centres.

The syndromes selected by the WHO for syndromic surveillance are: urethral discharge and genital ulceration. These two syndromes better reflect the incidence of STIs in the context of programme management in a given area or country.

Service providers :

- health agents ;
- community health workers.

Equipment :

- consultation register ;
- NOTIFICATION FORM ;
- support from the national health information service.

Periodicity: continuous throughout the year.

Target groups/beneficiaries: all patients with 1ST and their partners.

- Prevalence study

This is a study which consists of determining the proportion of existing cases of STIs (old and new cases) in a population at a given time.

Service providers :

- health agents ;
- statistics and epidemiology unit staff ;
- biologists ;
- laboratory technicians.

Equipment :

- consultation register ;
- notices ;
- survey protocols ;
- laboratory equipment and products
- reports from the national health information service

Periodicity :

Every year (as part of the annual production of activities)

Target groups / beneficiaries

Representative sample of the population.

- Monitoring the etiology of syndromes

This study is used to determine the most common causes of STI syndromes.

The syndromes to be studied are :

- urethral flow ;
- vaginal discharge ;
- genital ulceration.

Service providers :

- doctors, midwives, nurses ;
- statistics and epidemiology unit staff ;
- biologists ;
- laboratory technicians.

Equipment :

- survey protocol ;
- laboratory equipment and products.

Periodicity: every 3 - 5 years.

Target groups/beneficiaries: all patients with 1ST and their partners.

- Monitoring antibiotic resistance

This activity is used to determine the sensitivity of germs to the most common antibiotics for STI syndromes.

The germs to watch out for are : *Neisseria gonorrheae; Chlamydia trachomatis; Haemophilus*

ducreyi; Mycoplasma genitalium, Mycoplasma hominis.
Service providers:
- doctors ;
- statistics and epidemiology unit staff ;
- biologists ;
- laboratory technicians.

Equipment :
- survey protocol ;
- laboratories ;
- laboratory equipment and products required.

Periodicity: every 3 - 5 years
Target groups/beneficiaries: all patients with an STI and their partners.
- Special studies

The special studies provide scientific evidence and strategic information for implementing and evaluating the effectiveness of the 1ST Programme.
The main special studies are :
- trend study ;
- evaluation of algorithms ;
- seroprevalence survey (syphilis, HIV);
- incidence and prevalence of complications ;
- prevalence and causes of persistent urethritis ;
- study of risk factors
- studies of prevalence in certain vulnerable groups ;
- study of the costs of treating 1ST ;
- study of the quality of services offered and patient or population satisfaction
- behaviour monitoring.

Table 22: Standards for epidemiological surveillance of 1ST

SERVICE/ ACTIVITY	SERVICE SUPPLIERS				PERIODICITY	TARGET GROUPS/ BENEFICIARIES
	Biologist	Staff of the epidemiology and statistics units	Nurse / Midwife	Doctor		
Syndromic notification	+	+	+	+	Continuous monitoring (all year round)	Patients with 1ST and their partners
Prevalence study	+	+	+	+	Tons for 3-5 year olds	Representative sample of the population
Monitoring the etiology of syndromes	+	+	+	+	Tons for 3-5 year olds	Tons patients with 1ST and their partners
Monitoring antibiotic resistance	+	+	+	+	Tons for 3-5 year olds	Tons patients with 1ST and their partners

*4.6.2. **Procedures***

- **Syndromic notification of 1ST**

To carry out syndromic surveillance, you need :
- data collection ;
- data verification ;
- the initial analysis of data by the peripheral and intermediate levels;
- transmission of the data collected ;
- analysis at central level ;
- feedback ;

- disseminating information.

Data collection

Data is collected systematically, starting with the diagnosis, on the basis of accepted case definitions.

In first contact facilities, during routine consultations each provider must :

- regular and proper completion of the consultation register ;
- completing individual and weekly summary forms ;
- regular analysis of the data collected ;
- produce a monthly report ;
- draw up reports in duplicate (one copy for the hierarchical level and one copy for the health facility's archives).

Whatever the level of the health pyramid, reports must be drawn up and forwarded to the hierarchical level within the prescribed time limits. It is important to keep an up-to-date table in the health facility showing the number of STI cases each month. Curves and diagrams updated each month can also be used.

Verification of the reliability of the data collected

At every level of the health pyramid, regular monitoring is needed to ensure the reliability of the data.

Data analysis at peripheral and intermediate levels

Data must be analysed at every level of :

- the care delivery structure ;
- the epidemiology or health statistics unit at peripheral level ;
- the intermediate-level epidemiology or health statistics unit.

Data transmission

Once completed, the notification forms can be transmitted using the most reliable and secure means: all means of communication (traditional road transport, if possible with the help of the community); post office vehicles, radio messages using the channels of the national gendarmerie, prefectoral services or any other sector, telephone, fax, Internet, etc.). At present, health services are increasingly digitised, with data being sent* electronically or entered directly into a database validated by all the parties involved.

Central data analysis

It is carried out by the national health information service, which receives the data from the intermediate level in collaboration with the STI programme monitoring and evaluation service. This department must ensure that all the collection and verification procedures have been carried out correctly.

At all levels, we need to ensure that the data is validated and complete. *Feedback*

This can be done during a supervisory visit or a coordination meeting. Each level of the pyramid must provide feedback to the level below.

Dissemination of information

It is done through :

- the periodic bulletin of national health statistics ;
- the national STI and HIV surveillance bulletin ;
- WHO periodic bulletins ;
- periodic review of programme activities with stakeholders
- scientific publications ;
- Programme or Ministry of Health websites
- **Monitoring the prevalence of 1ST**

To determine the prevalence of STIs, studies are usually carried out on populations that are regularly screened. Specifically designed studies are also used to obtain data that can be used for programme planning.

The various methodological aspects of monitoring the prevalence of STIs must be the subject of a duly written protocol based on well-defined standards.

- **Monitoring germ resistance to antibiotics**

In order to adapt 1ST treatments to the most effective drugs, a study of the resistance of germs to drugs is necessary (especially for gonococcus). To be carried out, this monitoring also requires the use of a protocol based on well-established standards.

- **Assessing the etiology of syndromes**

Robust study protocols with laboratory equipment should be developed (in collaboration with teams in countries with adequate technical facilities) to carry out the majority of etiological diagnoses of STIs, enabling the etiologies of syndromes to be assessed.

3.7. Management of medicines and medical inputs

In addition to the traditional components of the programme, there are support services for drug management, medical devices and laboratory inputs.

The management of medicines, medical devices and laboratory products is the set of provisions that govern the estimation of their need, their supply, storage, distribution and use. The aim of this management is to ensure the availability, quality and permanent accessibility of medicines, medical devices and laboratory products in health facilities, in accordance with standards.

- .7.1 Standards

Management tools

The tools used to manage drugs, medical devices and laboratory products are :

- list of medicines, medical devices and laboratory products ;
- prescription (counterfoil) ;
- daily receipts and payments book ;
- the reception booklet ;
- the stock management sheet ;
- the stock tracking sheet ;
- the inventory register ;
- the order form ;
- the complaints book ;
- IT management tools.

Service providers :

- Directors/Programme Managers ;
- pharmacists ;
- biologists ;
- laboratory technicians ;
- formal health agents ;
- other form agents.

Premises and equipment:

- premises suitable for the proper storage of medicines, medical devices and laboratory products ;
- suitable equipment.

Products to manage:

- STI drugs ;
- medical devices (condoms, contraceptives) ;
- laboratory products.
- Table 23: Standards for the management of medical inputs

ACTIVITIES	SERVICE SUPPLIERS			MANAGEMENT TOOLS
	Health Agents	Pharmacist Biologist Lab technician	Director	
1. Choice of	+	+	+	List of medicines, medical devices

medicines, medical devices and laboratory products				and laboratory products.
2. Quantification	+	+	+	Notification forms Activity report.
3. Sourcing	+	+	+	Stock tracking sheets, purchase orders.
4. Receipt of order	+	+	+	Delivery notes Invoices.
5. Storage	+	+	+	Stock management sheets Book of joumalieres receipts and payments.
6. Distribution	+	+	+	Orders Number of health facilities at all levels served.

3.7.2 *Procedures*

- **The order**
- Make a list of products to be ordered;
- Fill in the order form and send it by the specified date;
- Only order products for which the quantities in stock on the stock cards are less than or equal to the calculated alert threshold;
- Keep a copy of the order form, record and archive it.
- **Receipt of delivery**
- Check that all the packages mentioned on the packing slip have been delivered;
- Protect all parcels from heat, rain and theft;
- Opening parcels ;
- Group and count the products received with the duplicate order form;
- Compare the quantity and quality of the products delivered with the delivery note or invoice;
- Check the expiry dates of products received and the integrity of bottles and other breakable products;
- Enter the revised quantities and the delivery note number on the stock sheets;
- Enter the value of stock received;
- Keep a chronological archive of supporting documents for entries.
- **Storage**
- Arrange products on shelves, taking into account the expiry date of products received and products already in stock;
- Store products away from heat, damp, rain, rodents and insects.
- **Selling products to patients**
- Deliver medicines on presentation of an invoiced prescription written by a prescriber approved by the health facility;
- Cash in the corresponding amount ;
- Keep a copy of the prescription-invoice;
- Record the products dispensed on a tally sheet or enter them directly on the stock sheets as they leave the pharmacy, depending on the pharmacy's internal organisation.
- Stock records must be updated on a daily basis, with the quantities of each product delivered recorded on the output side and the destination "sale to patient" indicated;
- **Removal for loss, damage or breakage**
- Remove the products from the shelves, record the removals on the corresponding stock sheets and write "loss/damage/breakage" in the "observation" column;
- Store lost, damaged or broken products in a special crate or on a shelf reserved for this purpose;

- Record these products in a "loss/damage/breakage" notebook;
- Periodically prepare a final stock withdrawal statement ;
- Return the damaged or broken products to the person in charge of their destruction against the duly signed report;
- Enter the number and date of the final issue report in the "observation" column corresponding to the stock records of the products concerned.
- **Inventory**
- Carry out a periodic inventory at least twice a year;
- Valuing stock on the basis of inventory results;
- Drawing up the pharmacy's financial statements.
- **Preventing out-of-stock situations**
- Process a command as soon as the alert threshold is reached.
- Notify the site manager and prescribers of any stock shortages.

Pa threshold p'alertd is /<? level Pa slock p above which it is necessary to trigger an order to avoid a shortage. It is also known as critical stock or alarm stock.

Calculation method

The alert threshold, which tells the manager when to trigger the order, is calculated on the basis of average daily consumption.

[S'H = .S'. .S' *(IC M CMM(+ (DL X CMM)*

SA = alert threshold

SS = safety threshold = CMM x DL/2

CMM = average monthly consumption = output over 1 year/12 months

DL = delivery time in months

CI = commcmde interval ep months

References

1. World Health Organization. Sexually transmitted infections and other reproductive tract infections. Essential practices guide. Geneva 2005
2. World Health Organization. Global strategy for the control of sexually transmitted infections. WHO Geneva 2006
3. Steen R, Elvira T, Kamali A et al. Control of sexually transmitted infections and prevention of HIV transmission: mending a fractured paradigm. Bull World Health Org 2009; 87: 858-65
4. Mayaud P, Mabey D. Approaches to the control of sexually transmitted infections in developing countries: old problems and modern challenges Sex Transm Infect 2004 ;80:174-82
5. Grosskurth H, Mwijarubi E, Todd J et al. Operational performance of an STD control programme in Mwanza Region, Tanzania. Sex Transm Infect 2000;76:426-36.
6. Bosch-Capblanch X, Liaqat S, Garner P. Managerial supervision to improve primary health care in low- and middle-income countries.Cochrane Database Syst Rev 2011 Sep 7;2011(9):CD006413. doi: 10.1002/14651858.CD006413.pub2.
7. Programme national de lutte contre le Sida et les 1ST, ministere de la sante du Togo. Guide de prise en charge des IST, 2015.
8. JHPIEGO. Family Health and AIDS Prevention Project. Normes et procedures pour la prise en charge des IST. General document for West and Central Africa April 2002. 97 pages
9. Togo Ministry of Health. Programme National de Lutte contre le Sida et les IST. Normes et procedures en matiere de pris en charge des IST, 2006, 83 pages
10. National AIDS and STI control programme (Togo). Normes, procedure en matiere de conseil et depistage. 2010, 78 pages
11. National programme to combat AIDS and STIs (Cote d'Ivoire). Standards and procedures for the management of STIs, 2015

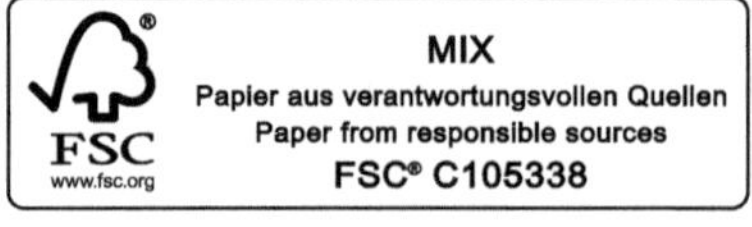

Printed by Books on Demand GmbH, Norderstedt / Germany